Learning Skills for Nursing Students

Nicola Davis, Alison C Clark,
Martina O'Brien, Caroline Plaice,
Karen Sumpton and Suzanne Waugh

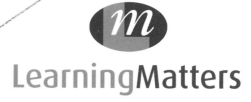

LearningMatters

First published in 2011 by Learning Matters Ltd

British Library Cataloguing in Publication Data
A CIP record for this book is available from the British Library

ISBN: 978 1 84445 376 4

This book is also available in the following ebook formats:

Adobe ebook: 978 1 84445 765 6
ePUB ebook: 978 1 84445 764 9
Kindle: 978 0 85725 023 0

Cover and text design by Toucan Design
Project management by Diana Chambers
Typeset by Kelly Winter
Printed and bound in Great Britain by Short Run Press, Exeter, Devon

Learning Matters Ltd
20 Cathedral Yard
Exeter EX1 1HB
Tel: 01392 215560
E-mail: info@learningmatters.co.uk
www.learningmatters.co.uk

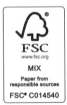

FSC
www.fsc.org
MIX
Paper from
responsible sources
FSC® C014540

Contents

About the authors

Nicola Davis is a Senior Lecturer in the Faculty of Health and Life Sciences at the University of the West of England, where she teaches and researches on interprofessional working, work-based learning and evidence-based care. An experienced registered nurse, she has worked in critical care, general medical nursing, research and staff development within the NHS.

Alison C Clark is a Lecturer in the School of Nursing, Midwifery and Physiotherapy at the University of Nottingham. She teaches across nursing theory and practice with a specific remit for public health and health promotion, and also teaches health psychology, professional development and mentorship.

Martina O'Brien is Senior Lecturer in Adult Nursing at London South Bank University, where she teaches on pre-registration courses. Martina's clinical nursing background is mainly in surgical nursing and practice development. The units of study she has responsibility for include medicines management and professional role development for adult branch nurses.

Caroline Plaice is Faculty Librarian in the Faculty of Health and Life Sciences at the University of the West of England where she leads a library team providing resources and support to students, staff and health professionals.

Karen Sumpton is a Digital Skills Trainer at the University of Salford. Her background is in librarianship and IT training. She currently runs the ECDL programme and provides training in a wide range of IT software and learning technologies.

Suzanne Waugh is Learning Skills Tutor at the University of Salford. Her background is in both Archaeology and Psychology, and she currently runs the University's study skills programme. Suzanne is also a qualified adult numeracy teacher, and is developing numeracy provision for student nurses.

Acknowledgements

The authors and publisher wish to thank the University of the West of England, Bristol, for their kind permission to give access to their interactive internet-based information literacy package (iSkillZone) produced by Library staff as an exemplar in Chapter 7 of the virtual resources libraries can provide, and for the screen shots of the library catalogue in Figures 7.1, 7.4 and 7.5. Driscoll's model of reflection (Figure 9.1) is taken from Chapter 2: Supported reflective learning: the essence of clinical supervision?, published in Driscoll, J J (ed.) (2007) *Practising Clinical Supervision: A reflective approach for healthcare professionals* (2nd edition). Edinburgh: Bailliere Tindall. Copyright Elsevier; reproduced by kind permission of Elsevier. Gibbs' model of reflection (Figure 9.2) is taken from Gibbs, G (1988) *Learning by Doing: A Guide to Teaching and Learning Methods*. Oxford: Further Education Unit, Oxford Brookes University. Copyright Oxford Brookes University; reproduced by kind permission of Oxford Brookes University. Johns' model of structured reflection (Table 9.1) is taken from Johns, C (2004) *Becoming a Reflective Practitioner* (2nd edition). Oxford: Wiley Blackwell. Copyright John Wiley and Sons Ltd; reproduced by kind permission of John Wiley and Sons Ltd.

Introduction

What to expect from this book

This book will introduce you to the key transferable, intellectual and graduate skills that you need to develop as you prepare to be a nurse. These crucial skills underpin your personal and professional development, both throughout your programme and as a registered nurse, and provide a solid base for lifelong learning. The book is designed primarily for first-year nursing students following any of the pre-registration fields of practice, but it may also be very helpful to students or nurses who need to refresh any of the main learning skills.

Book structure

The book begins with a welcoming first chapter that introduces you to nursing education and what you can expect from your course of study. In this chapter you will be presented with some of the key issues to consider as you commence your learning journey, while preparing to become a registered nurse. It is very important to consider what you expect of yourself as a learner, what you expect of your course and what will be expected of you.

In Chapter 2, Suzanne Waugh presents an overview of some of the basic study and writing skills you need to refine. These include time management, self-management, note-taking in lectures and from sources, how to write assignments and make your arguments more convincing, how to tackle exams and how to prepare for placements.

Chapter 3, written by Martina O'Brien, focuses on 'being numerate'. This is clearly an essential skill in terms of preparing to administer medications. However, being numerate also helps you to be competent in delivering many aspects of nursing care. It is therefore timely to revise the principles of maths related to nursing during this early stage and concentrate on the important numerical skills you will be using throughout your course and specifically in nursing practice.

In Chapter 4 you are introduced to the vital issue of developing interpersonal skills. Nursing inevitably involves working with people. When working with service users, patients and other healthcare professionals, being able to communicate effectively is absolutely essential to the establishment of the therapeutic relationship. It involves developing insight into the impact of both verbal and non-verbal cues. This is also integral to interprofessional teamwork.

In Chapter 5 Alison C Clark focuses on the essential skill of literacy, helping you to further develop the basic writing skills introduced in Chapter 2. It is crucial to be able to write clearly and well in order to succeed in both writing assignments about nursing issues and in delivering care. This chapter focuses on the latter – what forms of written information are used in practice (for example, care plans and records, information for patients, referrals and handovers, reports), to whom they are addressed (for example, patients and service users, other team members, senior management and professional organisations) and how to write successfully for these various audiences. You also need to be able to record your development, demonstrate your knowledge and understanding, as well as most importantly documenting the care that you give.

Within Chapter 6 Karen Sumpton sets out the increasing range of information technology skills that are expected of nursing students, and guides you in developing your IT skills. This is of great benefit for both theory and practice. Practice is evolving and needs to be proactive in maximising the potential offered within the digital age.

Within Chapter 7 the importance of information literacy is considered. What it is, what it involves and how to get the very best service from your library is integral to the consideration of this essential skill. At this stage in your studies, you may not realise exactly how much the library can do to help you in terms of study skills and information retrieval. This is also a key skill in practice, which will help you keep up to date with the latest research and evidence bases.

Chapter 8 follows logically from the previous chapter and introduces you to the skills needed for evidence-based practice (EBP) in addition to information literacy. Within this chapter, EBP is defined, types of sources of evidence are considered and the fundamental building blocks of constructing a critical appraisal of these main types of sources are discussed. Imperative to EBP is the inclusion of, and working in partnership with, patients and informal carers.

Chapter 9 deals with the important skill of reflection, both in practice and afterwards, which is so important in the development of competence in nursing. This chapter explores what reflection is, how it can help your practice and how you might find it better supported with the use of an established model of reflection. It is vital to see this as an integral part of self-development.

Finally, building on important points made within the previous chapter, Chapter 10 helps you to consider how to build your personal development plan, within a formal portfolio. This can become a vital record of your learning and practice, which should help you to develop during your studies and also start on the career pathway you chose for yourself at the end of your studies.

This book is intended as an introduction to each of the learning skills presented, and will hopefully provide you with a good framework from which to explore and learn further. You will be expected to read more widely and the further reading and useful website suggestions at the end of each chapter should give you a useful starting point for further study. Words in **bold** appear in the Glossary on page 212.

Nursing offers you tremendous career opportunities, in many diverse areas of practice. Nurses and nursing offers an invaluable service when it is done well. We hope that this book helps to engage you in developing a sustained passion for delivering safe and effective care, in partnership with all those people who you care for, as well as enjoying your learning journey right from the very beginning.

Chapter 1
Beginning your learning in nursing
Nicola Davis

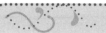 **NMC Standards for Pre-registration Nursing Education**

This chapter will address the following competencies:

Domain 1: Professional values

1. All nurses must practise with confidence according to *The Code: Standards of conduct, performance and ethics for nurses and midwives* (NMC 2008b), and within other recognised ethical and legal frameworks. They must be able to recognise and address ethical challenges relating to people's choices and decision-making about their care, and act within the law to help them and their families and carers find acceptable solutions.

7. All nurses must be responsible and accountable for keeping their knowledge and skills up to date through continuing professional development. They must aim to improve their performance and enhance the safety and quality of care through evaluation, supervision and appraisal.

Domain 4: Leadership, management and team working

4. All nurses must be self-aware and recognise how their own values, principles and assumptions may affect their practice. They must maintain their own personal and professional development, learning from experience, through supervision, feedback, reflection and evaluation.

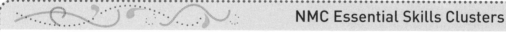 **NMC Essential Skills Clusters**

This chapter will prepare you for the chapters that follow, which focus on specific ESCs.

Chapter aims

By the end of this chapter, you should understand:

- some of the key expectations of you as a student at university;
- the need to be an effective independent learner and some of the learning challenges you may face;

- expectations of nursing students in particular, such as professional suitability and behaviour;
- why the Nursing and Midwifery Council regulates nurses and nursing students.

Introduction

Within this chapter we will consider what it means to be a nursing student, who you are as a learner and where that places you as you begin your nursing studies. Your university will have specific expectations of you as a student. You may also have lots of ideas about what to expect from your nursing course, some of which will be right, others of which may be challenged along the way. One of the hardest things to grasp for many new students is that higher education requires you to be an independent learner. This may involve challenging yourself in terms of where, how and for how long you can study by yourself. There will be support and advice available, but also the expectation that you will 'take the reins' and manage yourself as a self-motivated student. You will also have to learn how to be proactive, self-evaluative and reflective in your learning, and be honest with yourself about when it is time to ask for help. The first half of this chapter guides you through some of the challenges you may face as you start your nursing training, and helps you to assess your expectations and abilities as a learner.

You will also find that being a nursing student differs in many ways from being a student on other higher education courses. Even before you commenced your nursing studies you may have had ideas about what preparing to be a nurse might involve and include. As you progress through the course you might find that some of these expectations are met easily but others might surprise you, such as the importance placed on how you behave in your personal life. You will be learning in practice, in a variety of clinical environments, in contact with patients, service users and many other healthcare professionals, and you will be expected to behave as a responsible professional, even before you qualify. Therefore, the second half of the chapter helps you to understand the general expectations of nursing students in terms of behaviour, professional conduct and performance, and how this relates to the Nursing and Midwifery Council's (NMC) main function in regulating nursing. We will also highlight why learning skills, such as those covered in this book, are fundamental to practising as a nurse and not just of use for your years as a student. You will need to recognise, appreciate and develop all of these key transferable skills in order to succeed in professional nursing practice.

What is expected of university study?

Your past experiences of learning might include being at school where the tasks required of you were very specific and the material you needed to know made readily available. You may also have experienced learning within further education where you were expected to become a more independent learner, yet still had a very full and structured week. Indeed, you may have worked in part-time or full-time employment, which will have enhanced a number of specific skills. You will notice right from the beginning of the course how diverse your cohort is, representing a great range of individual students with different backgrounds. You need to evaluate where your past experience places you in terms of building on those skills and attributes for the future. Beginning a course at university will involve many opportunities and challenges. Staff will be available to help you with specific issues like study skills, self-management and even pastoral support. Whatever your past experiences, it is very important to remember that you already have strengths: you achieved the entry criteria for your course and you passed the selection process. So the foundation is there for you to build on. Let's start the process with a small activity designed to help you celebrate the strengths that you already possess.

Activity 1.1   *Reflection*

Either on paper or electronically, create a new document with the title 'My Strengths'. On this page, which you can display at home, record your thoughts on what skills, experiences and attributes you think are going to help you during your nursing studies. Put this either in a list form or scattered across the page. Do this in one bright colour. Return to this page on several occasions during your studies, and with a different colour pen record how you are developing your knowledge, understanding and skills. You might also like to think about how some of the skills 'join-up' – for example, both effective communication and writing contribute equally well to the requirement to document nursing care.

An outline answer is provided at the end of the chapter.

What is meant by independent learning?

Whatever your learning experiences so far, at university you will be expected to take the lead responsibility for your own learning and development. After all, you are the person who knows best where you are in terms of your level of understanding and intellectual skills. Being an independent learner means three things:

* understanding your learning needs: what current knowledge and skills you have and what you need to develop;
* understanding your learning style: what type of learner you are and how that influences both where and how you learn best;
* being motivated to engage in a significant amount of self-study on your own, and identify when you need extra support and follow that through with appropriate action.

The university's expectations will be made clear to you when you commence your studies: you may not be required to be in class all day or every day, even when you are doing theory modules. The university will expect you to be self-motivated enough to take your own learning forward by making an honest assessment of your learning needs and what type of learner you are, and then by getting on and doing the learning.

Your learning needs

Activity 1.1 is a good starting point for consciously thinking about and assessing your learning needs. You should have identified strengths that you can build on already, and the next step in the process is to identify areas where you need to develop your knowledge and skills. In order to do this, you first have to work out what knowledge and skills you need to have. Being very clear about what will be involved in your studies will help you to make realistic and achievable plans.

In Chapter 10 we will consider how the compilation of a portfolio, including a personal development plan, is very useful in helping you to plot out your baseline and developing skills. You may be given a portfolio when you commence your studies, which you may share with mentors in practice and have reviewed by your personal tutor. View this as an essential resource, in which a record of your achievements is kept safe, secure and close to hand.

Understanding your course requirements

Once you commence your studies you will be given information in your programme handbooks, which might cover quite a broad range. If you are following a modular programme you will also be given module handbooks. These will include the learning outcomes that you will need to address and may be assessed on. Amid this plethora of information you will need to map out what you expect of yourself, what the course expects of you and how you can develop yourself in order to meet those expectations. You need to be very clear about what the different assessments you need to undertake actually focus on and involve. Thoroughly reading the material that you are given on the course, as well as checking out your understanding with your tutors, should help you find clarity and hopefully achieve well.

Assessment of where you want your career to take you

Your course may well be one of the major landmarks in your life's adventure, but be mindful of your destination. The years will go by very quickly and in a very short amount of time you may be looking for your first nursing post. Thinking about where you want to be in the future right at the start of your studies will help you assess your learning needs and strengths and weaknesses against a specific aim. This will also make your learning needs assessment much more meaningful and will keep you motivated.

Through your theory and practice modules, reflect on what aspects of nursing interest you most and how you might develop yourself to work effectively within specific clinical areas in the future. You might not know exactly which area of nursing that you want to aim for right now. However, you may develop insight into what particular specialities interest you during the course. For example, you might decide that you want to work in theatre because you like working within set routines and are interested in supporting patients through such an acute experience. Or you might be attracted to the high level of partnership working around health education within primary care. The variety of practice experiences that you encounter will give you the opportunity to learn specific skills and consider whether you enjoy a particular type of nursing. Reflect on these experiences well, really capitalise on those learning opportunities and write about them in the personal section of your portfolio.

Thinking about your potential career destination from the start of your studies will also make you more employable in the future. Employers will appreciate that you have put thought into your chosen career, have self-assessed your abilities against the role, and developed weaker areas of your skills profile. In a job interview, you may be asked where you see yourself in three, five or ten years' time, so this process of thinking about your future and assessing your skills against this will also help you during interviews. Your university may hold specific sessions to get you thinking about how marketable you are now and could be in the future, so make full use of these opportunities. Employers will have specific expectations of what they require of employees in terms of core and transferable skills, so looking at job adverts in similar roles will help you gain an insight into your chosen career. You might also want to look at the NHS Knowledge and Skills Framework and Skills for Health Competencies for the role, if applicable, at **https://tools.skillsforhealth.org.uk**.

Activity 1.2   *Reflection*

Either on paper or electronically, create a new document with the title 'What an employer might expect of me'. Record your thoughts on what skills, experiences and attributes you think an employer might need and value. Put this either in a list or scattered across the page. Do this in one bright colour. Return to this page on several occasions during your studies and with a different colour pen make a record of how you are developing your knowledge, understanding and skills in order to match those expectations. You will need to be both creative and proactive in how you market yourself in the future.

An outline answer is provided at the end of the chapter.

Transferable skills

Any higher education qualifications you have will serve you well if they are augmented by clear mastery of all of the key transferable skills discussed in this book, so you should plot your learning needs for these too. In your first year of study there may be specific sessions on numeracy, information literacy, information technology and interpersonal skills, all transferable skills that are vital within nursing practice and expected by the NMC at point of registration (we will explore the reasons for this later in the chapter).

What type of learner are you?

Cottrell (2003, p4) advises that we can:

use many senses . . . The more we use our senses of sight, hearing and touch, and the more we use fine muscle movement in looking, speaking, writing, typing, drawing, or moving the body, the more opportunities we give the brain to take in information using our preferred sense.

As Cottrell is suggesting here, there are many ways to learn, and you need to think about what methods of learning might be most meaningful to you.

Activity 1.3   *Critical thinking*

Start by thinking about how you like to learn now. You might think that you are quite a passive learner and like to sit in a lecture hall and just listen or take notes. Similarly, you might feel that you need structure to your learning and prefer specific instructions. However, this may be because your learning experiences so far have encouraged these methods of learning. You might find it easier to take in and retain information if you read quietly on your own, or you might learn more effectively in a group. There are several online self-evaluation tools that you can use in order to develop your insight into this aspect of yourself. One example of these is the VARK guide to learning styles, available at **www.vark-learn.com/english/index.asp.**

An outline answer is provided at the end of the chapter.

Once you have gained insight into your learning preferences or styles, you can adapt to make the very best use of learning opportunities within a variety of contexts, but be prepared to be flexible. Cottrell (2003) advises that whether you discover that you have a type or not, it may change because we are adaptable creatures. In addition, nursing courses tend to be defined by the diversity of the content and methods of learning. You need to be prepared to learn in more than one way. You may think that nursing is best learnt in practice, but that is only partly correct. Preparing for learning in practice by undertaking other types of learning, such as reading the underpinning theory or context for an area of practice, will help you make the most of such experiences. (Chapter 8, pages 166–7, explores the practice-based aspect of learning in more detail, as does another book in this series: *Successful Practice Learning for Nursing Students*, Sharples, 2011).

Learning challenges and keeping motivated

As we have already highlighted, doing a significant amount of self-study might not be something that you have been used to before. You may find it challenging to be faced with a vast amount of reading and assignments with no guidance about where to start. Chapter 2 helps you to master some basic study skills that will help you to feel more confident about where to start and what is expected of you. In order to keep motivated throughout your learning, it is also a good idea to think about the challenges you may face and the strategies you will need to deal with them. Let's look at some of the common challenges that nursing students can face and how you might prepare for them.

Feeling isolated

When you arrive at university for the first time you may be struck by the large size of the campus. For the first year you may also be living on or very near the campus and so most of your time may be spent in this new environment. You may feel anxious as to whether you are going to make new friends or whether you will now have the time to keep in contact with old friends. You might feel overwhelmed at first by the amount there is to learn and not know where to start.

It is therefore important to remember that you will not be alone at the forefront of directing your own learning. You will be part of a cohort and be allocated to smaller groups within that large cohort. Your personal tutor group may have between 20 and 30 students in it. You will find that you share many learning experiences in that group and this may help to enable peer supported learning (as explored further in Chapter 4). Social networking sites and informal study groups help in developing social connections and new friends as well as learning in a way that is comfortable for you. The benefit of being on campus is its social and educational opportunities. Take advantage of the full student experience when you commence the course, including capitalising on opportunities to spend time with others who share your specific interests.

Finding sources of support

There should be specific staff at your university who can offer formal student advice on financial issues, put you in touch with emotional support or help you to make contact with study skills advisers. If you feel that you need a specific assessment of your learning needs, there may be specific student advisers on campus who can facilitate that. It is very important to feel that there are avenues of support and advice open to you. Your personal tutor should also be a source of individual and pastoral support. That particular member of staff should be well placed to support, review and advance your learning journey.

Time

At the start of your course you may think that you have plenty of time. However, time is a finite resource so you need to manage yourself in order to make the very best use of the time available. A great deal will be expected of you and there will be a lot of pressure on you and your time. You need to start planning your study schedule, plotting out when assignment submission dates are looming and being prepared. This may include plotting out how much time to allocate to each component of study, building up to the completion of those assignments. Build in some slippage time as non-achievement can be very demotivating. Remember that it is unlikely that you will ever find the perfect day to study; it's far more likely that you will find small snippets of time every so often when it is possible to study, so take this into account when you are planning. There is specific advice on time management in Chapter 2 (see pages 23–5).

The responsibilities of the nursing student

Earlier in this chapter we discussed the importance of considering your employability from the very first day of your course. Part of this will involve considering the standards of behaviour

expected of you, so we will move now from thinking about you as a learner to specifically considering you as a nursing student, who will also need to perform well in practice.

You will probably be aware from attending selection events or open days that you will be learning
both in the university and within practice. These practice learning experiences are exciting,
challenging and fundamental to your studies, but you should also remember that there will be
specific expectations regarding how to behave as a nursing student. Even if you have worked as
a Healthcare Assistant (HCA) for years, you will now be learning how to be an effective student,
preparing towards becoming a registered nurse (RN). That is a very different role. The risk in
'over-selling' your experience as an HCA is that you just might find yourself being subsumed into
that role again, which will not help to refocus you on the new nursing role that you are there to
learn. At the same time, however, do not think that certain tasks are 'beneath you' as it is often
in the most mundane tasks, such as bed-bathing, that you get to understand the holistic needs of
those in your care. It is important to bear in mind that you will be supervised in practice by
experienced practitioners who should guide you through your first placement with particular
attention to your orientation to practice. Remember that you are supernumerary in practice. This
should enable you to make the best use of the learning opportunities during placements. There
will still be an expectation that you will be involved in delivering care, but this is in addition to
those who are directly employed to do so. The NMC issues guidance to nursing students to clarify
their position within practice, particularly affirming what you can and cannot be asked to do.
Chapters 8, 9 and 10 contain advice and activities that relate to the issues of nursing students'
rights and responsibilities. See also Sharples (2009) for a consideration of how you can succeed
in your practice learning.

On a practical note, you will need to be measured for a uniform for practice learning: make sure
that it is ordered in a size that looks professional and feels comfortable to work in for up to 12
hours at a stretch. In some practice learning opportunities you may not have to wear a uniform,
but remember that you are still expected to present yourself as a professional in the public eye,
and should dress appropriately. Ask your personal tutor or mentor in practice beforehand for
guidance if you are unsure about what is suitable.

You probably expected that your course would prepare you to be safe and professional in practice,
but might be quite surprised that you are also advised to maintain a high standard of conduct in
the university and in your personal life. Media depictions of rebellious, raucous and sometimes
erratic student behaviour may sit at odds with what you are currently being told about how to
behave on campus. This is because you are doing a programme that is NMC approved, preparing
you to be registered with the NMC. There are specific NMC expectations about the amount of
time that you will complete set curriculum content and expectations of working towards the
professional standard of conduct. We will consider this in the next section on accountability. You
should be mindful of the impression you convey, verbally and non-verbally, including the way
that you present yourself. Within the NMC *Code*, nurses are mandated to work co-operatively
within and beyond their own profession at all times. You will also be expected to learn co-
operatively with your peers, contributing to creating an environment in which you can all learn
effectively. Many of your co-students may become your work colleagues in the future. It will be
helpful to future working relationships if you have always made the effort to get on with your
peers. Always striving to professional behaviour will lay the foundations for an effective career.

Activity 1.4   *Reflection*

Think about the way that you currently present yourself in terms of how you dress, behave and socialise in public. How might you have to change these aspects of yourself when you are in practice?

An outline answer is provided at the end of the chapter.

You also need to consider how you present yourself in online environments (see also Chapter 6, pages 119–24). It is all too easy for very personal information to become very public on social networking sites and discussion forums, and disclosure of certain information could cause very real problems for you or others. It is also a requirement of the *NMC Guidance on Professional Conduct for Nursing and Midwifery Students* (NMC, 2010d) that you follow their advice on the use of social networking sites, which can be found on their website at **www.nmc-uk.org/Nurses-and-midwives/Advice-by-topic/A/Advice/Social-networking-sites**.

Scenario

Imagine that you had a really difficult day on your practice learning experience, and made a derogatory comment about your mentor on Facebook. Your mentor knows one of your friends on the site and sees your comment. A serious complaint is made against you at the university that jeopardises your future practice learning opportunities.

This scenario has already happened to a small number of students. The confidentiality of client information is paramount and you must not disclose it inappropriately via any medium, including online. You might also want to consider how carefully you need to make anonymous situations you have encountered in practice in order to maintain confidentiality when discussing them.

Activity 1.5   *Communication*

If you use a social networking site like Facebook, think about the type of information that you post. Do you talk about events that have occurred in placements or within your social life? Do you make comments about other people, some of which might be derogatory? Are you certain of who can and cannot access what you have said on these pages?

An outline answer is provided at the end of the chapter.

Many nursing students are being expected to sign up to professional standards in university contracts, even before registration, which demonstrates the responsibility inherent within the role from the very beginning.

Accountability

We have discussed above some key expectations of nursing students in terms of behaviour. We will now look a little deeper at why nurses and nursing students need to be responsible for their behaviour. Working towards a time when you may be registered with the NMC and therefore have full accountability, it is so important to behave in certain ways, to create the right impression.

Dimond (2004) offers expert insight into what she calls the four arenas of accountability, which are all relevant to the professional work of nurses. This accountability is asserted where there is an established duty of care, that is, the nurse is responsible for caring for a specific individual. The four arenas include the client, the public, the employer and the NMC. Where a duty of care is in place, the client has every right to expect the delivery of clinically effective nursing care. Should anything go wrong in terms of what is done to the client, or what has been missed, the client could sue the nurse responsible. If this breach caused serious physical harm or loss of life, this could then become a criminal matter, hence the potential for a public response. When a nurse is employed, rather than working as an independent practitioner (which is relatively rare), the employer requires that practice should be concordant with its policies and procedures. Should practice transgress these expectations, the client might sue the Trust employing the practitioner or the individual practitioner in civil court (Dimond, 2008). Under the former circumstances, the Trust may then terminate the nurse's contract because non-compliance with Trust policies would constitute a breach of contract with them. Arguably the highest level of expectation of professional conducts rests with accountability to the NMC. When a complaint is made against a registrant, the NMC will follow up the complaint and investigate. Should the complaint be upheld, the NMC can impose the ultimate sanction of taking the registrant off the register. So, bearing in mind all of these arenas of accountability the pressure to practise well is clearly high.

When you are in practice, the mentors who supervise you need to carefully consider the tasks that they delegate to you because they will remain accountable for the care that they delegate. As a nursing student, because you are not yet registered, the accountability has to rest with the registered staff on duty. When registered nurses delegate tasks that they are confident that the other person can complete, there is some mitigation. However, if an inappropriate task is delegated the accountability still rests squarely with the registered nurse. To do otherwise puts their employment and registration at risk. There may be a range of situations where you have to make difficult decisions when in practice. Let's consider a scenario where this occurs.

Scenario

Alex is a first-year nursing student in his first clinical placement. He is helping his mentor to bed bath an elderly patient. During this bed bath the elderly lady tells them both that one of the nurses on duty last night shouted at her because she kept pressing the call bell to ask for the commode. She says that several other patients on the ward are frightened of calling the bell at night because that particular nurse is 'bad tempered'. This elderly lady has a urinary tract infection and will understandably need to use the commode more often and she is also unable to walk to the toilet in time. Alex's mentor reassures the patient that she must call for assistance

continued opposite . . .

continued . . . .

when she needs it. However, after Alex has completed the bed bath and is clearing up in the sluice, he asks the mentor what should be done about what they have both been told. She says that the Ward Manager will have to be informed and that it will be his or her responsibility to make a decision about what action to take.

Recognising levels of competence

Within the scenario above, Alex the nursing student is working with his mentor. Alex is delivering care that he is developing confidence in and also being supervised to do so safely. However, the patient raises an issue that he would not be able to deal with on his own at this stage in his career.

Perhaps one of the most reasonable expectations of you, right from the beginning of your studies, is that you will be responsible only for practising those skills that you have been prepared for and therefore feel confident to carry out. Do bear in mind that any client has the right to refuse care given by a student, although they rarely exercise that right. What will help to reassure them is a clear demonstration that your practice is safe. Through developing your understanding, careful observation and appropriate levels of mentor supervision, you should securely progress your skills. In their standards for pre-registration education, the NMC set out specific expectations of skills and competence levels for each year of your course. At the beginning of every chapter following this one, the related Essential Skills Clusters and associated progression points will be highlighted.

Scenario

Felicia is a first-year student in her second clinical placement. She is asked by her mentor to take the morning medications to a patient on the other side of the ward who she has only met once. Felicia is worried about whether it is safe for her to do this. She is sure that she can remember being told at university that she cannot administer drugs on her own until she is registered. Does she have the time to ask anyone for advice?

Clinical governance

Clinical governance has transformed the expectation of the National Health Service (NHS) from one of needs-driven healthcare delivery to the requirement for consistently high standards of care and treatment. As with Health and Safety legislation, there are both individual and organisational requirements of clinical governance. Clinical governance was launched as a means to achieve the devolution of responsibility, combined with accountability for performance (Flynn, 2004). It asserts the centrality of the service user position, reinforcing their right to choose and direct their packages of care. The 'pillars' that support the structure representing clinical governance include effective risk management, patient liaison, research and development, complaints management and evidence-based practice (EBP). In the scenario above, Felicia clearly needs to consider the risks involved. This is because what the mentor has asked Felicia to do constitutes a 'near miss' as she is not in a position to engage in the lone administration of any medications. Should she just go ahead and do as the mentor suggests? If she did so, then she might give the medication to the wrong patient or in some other way contribute to a drug error, which could harm the patient and would require an incident form to be completed. In Chapter 8, related issues will be considered in more depth. This is important both legally as well as professionally, as discussed below.

Being a learning professional and the NMC

The above section considered the NMC role in terms of accountability and levels of competence. We will now explore that role in more detail and why regulation and accountability are so important throughout your course and beyond, moving into practice.

The Department of Health is clear in its assertion that nurses have a central co-ordinating role within the health service. Nurses are often the lead professionals co-ordinating complex packages of care that may involve effective liaison both within and beyond their own professional group. Nurses need to be effective at assessing care needs, planning care packages, delivering clinically effective care and evaluating the client response. All of these stages form the nursing process. Alongside this nurses need to be able to communicate effectively, act as advocates and develop themselves to keep their practice current. The proximity of nurses to the delivery of treatment and care, in terms of both quality and quantity, underlines how important it is that nursing practice is consistently judged to be worthy of public confidence. At the behest of government, the NMC seeks to ensure that this is exactly what happens; so it is an organisation that you need to be mindful of right from the beginning of your studies.

The NMC was formed in April 2002 as a regulatory body for nursing. Its main remit of ensuring public protection is maintained in several ways: through the enforcement of the *Code* of practice (NMC, 2008b) which all registered nurses must adhere to, through setting standards for pre-registration education and also through the wide dissemination of their advisory documentation. Your course will have been designed around the *Standards for Pre-registration Nursing Education* (NMC, 2010c), and there are specific competencies and skills it lists which you will be expected to have in order to register as a nurse at the end of your course. Education does not, however, end with your pre-registration training, as is made clear by the *Code*:

> *Keep your skills and knowledge up to date*
> - *38. You must have the knowledge and skills for safe and effective practice when working without direct supervision*
> - *39. You must recognise and work within the limits of your competence*
> - *40. You must keep your knowledge and skills up to date throughout your working life*
> - *41. You must take part in appropriate learning and practice activities that maintain and develop your competence and performance*

Therefore, the learning skills you develop as part of your programme, and as covered by this book, will prepare you for being a learning professional throughout your working life. The NMC makes clear that lifelong learning and contributing to an effective learning environment is every registered nurse's business.

Why is nursing regulated so rigorously by the NMC?

Every client in the community, just like every patient in a hospital ward, should feel confident of receiving safe and clinically effective care from any registered nurse. Inspiring and delivering on this expectation is vital in order to assert the professional status of nursing, which should offer a level of service that can be seen to be reliable, current and responsive. All service users are potentially vulnerable people and the 'safeguarding' agenda is a key priority for all healthcare professionals. Nurses are, by the very nature of their work, often caring directly for clients who are ill and therefore in a disempowered position. So all nurses need to be sensitive in their practice at all times. Nurses can also be involved in assessing situations where they might identify areas of risk to clients from family or specific activities in which the client might be engaged. Dealing with such issues requires the utmost tact and diplomacy. It is useful to see nursing as offering a service, with patients as consumers of that service. Whether they realise it or not, patients have rights, and perhaps especially if they do not realise this, nurses need to place themselves in a position to recognise and respect those rights.

Activity 1.6   *Reflection*

Have you ever been very ill? If not, talk to a friend, family member or fellow student who has been ill, and discuss their experiences with them (make sure they are willing to share information and be careful not to ask them to divulge anything they are not comfortable discussing with you). How did it make you/them feel? How did they feel about those caring for them? Consider writing a reflective account of this and putting it in your student portfolio.

An outline answer is provided at the end of the chapter.

Activity 1.6 should lead you to reflect on how important it is that those responsible for caring for ill and vulnerable people are appropriately trained and regulated and why the NMC's function in doing this is critically important. The NMC *Code* of professional conduct clearly sets out how nurses can inspire and earn public confidence, primarily by acting in the individual's best interests. This may involve:

- listening clearly to what the client wants, expects or needs;
- finding the appropriate resources with which to meet those needs;
- making referrals to other healthcare professionals;
- negotiating a compromise situation if there are insufficient resources to meet the client's requests.

Delivering care should always involve the assertion of fundamental respect for the individual and advocacy for the protection of their right to safe care. This situation might, however, be complicated further if the client has unrealistic or unsafe wants or needs. Consider the following scenario.

> ### Scenario
>
> *Mary is on her second clinical placement on a surgical ward and has been allocated to look after a young female patient who has a history of self-harm. This patient has been admitted for intravenous antibiotics and dressings to deep, infected wounds on both arms. Mary has been advised to monitor this young patient very carefully and stay with her when she goes to the bathroom. However, the young lady is becoming increasingly distressed that she cannot go the toilet on her own and is starting to become verbally aggressive.*

The above scenario reveals a real aspect of complexity in practice. Sometimes the clients we care for will have very different agendas from the ones that we imagine they might have. Not all clients want to follow a pathway that we advise or even quietly 'approve' of. Under such circumstances it is vital not to be seen to be judgemental. Nurses should place themselves in a position to deliver care using a conventional nursing process rather than a position where they decide whether the client deserves to be cared for. Mary will certainly need to consult with her mentor or one of the other registered nurses on the ward in order to alert them to developments within this situation. The patient should have been referred to the mental health team and this referral may need to become urgent. Mary will certainly need to be well supported by her mentor. This may be one of the cases that they can discuss in interim meetings; there is so much to learn about offering complex packages of care that may involve several different healthcare professionals.

The NMC and ethical principles

The NMC *Code*, and the Standards of Education, are clearly linked to fundamental ethical principles. The most prominent consideration is the duty of care as discussed on page 12. We will now look at some other key ethical principles that underpin nursing care, so that you can understand why the requirements for your professional behaviour are so important, even while you are a student. These principles should underpin all nursing knowledge and skills, including the learning skills covered by this book.

Beneficence and non-maleficence

Where there is a stated therapeutic relationship and once a duty of care is in place, nurses are expected to act in the individual service user or patient's best interests. This expectation can be linked to the fundamental ethical principle of beneficence or 'doing good'. This may involve delivering evidence-based practice or might involve advocating for an alternative course of action in response to individual choices. Nurses are also reminded through NMC regulation that the care they offer may also be judged not just in terms of what they do but also of what they do not do, legally regarded as 'omissions'. There is also the fundamental concept of non-maleficence or aspiring to 'do no harm'. Nurses should be mindful of the potential harm that could be a consequence of forgetting some aspect of care, which could be regarded as negligence. For example, if effective mouth care was not offered to a patient who needed it, then demineralisation of the teeth would incur damage that only a dental hygienist could resolve. Through one small omission, very real damage could occur. In addition, the patient who is not offered mouth care may feel very uncomfortable and self-conscious.

Recognising capacity in patients

The nurse operating as an effective advocate recognises and respects the position of clients and how defending their autonomy (the medical ethical principle of respecting the individual's right to make their own decisions and choices) is fundamentally important. The Mental Capacity Act (2005) requires all healthcare professionals to assess the capacity of all clients to make decisions for themselves. The Act makes allowance for the fact that the establishment of capacity can fluctuate. In our demographically ageing society, the number of older adults with cognitive impairment is also increasing. So nurses need to be prepared regularly to assess capacity and be prepared to work particularly hard to advocate for clients where they may have fluctuating levels of lucidity, affecting their mental capacity to make decisions for themselves.

Veracity and truthfulness

Perhaps one of the fundamental ethical principles that you may not have been aware of before is that of veracity or truthfulness: principles that are very reasonable expectations of nurses.

Scenario

Beth is a community nurse with two service users on her caseload who live next door to each other. Both consider themselves to be Beth's priority. In reality, both clients have an equal level of need and Beth has to decide who to visit first. If this situation stays stable and the visits go on long term, Beth has decided to be open and honest with both individuals and say that she will alternate who she visits first every week. The individual service users may now respect the fact that their expectations are being effectively managed and realise that Beth cannot be in two places at the same time.

Veracity is also very important when managing patient expectations as to when they will be attended to. How often do we hear of nurses saying they will 'be back in a minute' and then returning either hours afterwards or not at all? This behaviour may not be intentionally dishonest but it threatens the nurse–patient relationship. Telling the truth demonstrates a fundamental respect for the client.

Conclusion

You might be surprised to find the first chapter on a book on learning and study skills has such an emphasis on professionalism and the role of the nurse. You will now be starting to realise how learning skills are fundamental to being a professional and why it is so important to be an independent learner and practitioner. Learning skills such as those covered in this book are key transferable skills that will underpin every aspect of your practice. This includes how to communicate effectively, which will be discussed in more detail in Chapter 4 on interpersonal skills. Aspiring to be an effective communicator at all times will help you to build working and therapeutic relationships. As so much of the documentation of care may happen via computerised records, it is also important that you continue to develop your information technology and literacy skills. Preparing for the administration of medication will be one of the very real reasons why reinforcing your numeracy knowledge will be imperative. Acting in the best interests of clients and protecting your position of accountability will involve information literacy skills in order to start you on the stages of evidence-based practice. As you progress through this book, each chapter will take you through some of the fundamental aspects of all of these skills, signposting important concepts, key learning activities and relevant further reading.

Chapter summary

This chapter has introduced you to ways of managing yourself as an independent learner at university and within practice, and to what it means to be a learning professional within nursing. We first considered the expectations for university study and that as you take the lead responsibility for your own learning, you need to build on your strengths and capitalise on your capacity to develop yourself. The chapter looked briefly at some learning challenges, such as working with others and time management, which other chapters will return to in more depth.

We then turned to the specific expectations and responsibilities of the nursing student, and explored how these differ from other students. We outlined the expectations regarding professional behaviour at all times and why this is the case. Key to this is the notion of accountability, competence and the central importance of caring for and offering a service to the patient or client. Accountability also relates to clinical governance, which requires standardisation of quality care delivery with both individual and organisational responsibilities, and so we touched on this briefly. This chapter has considered some of the implications for registered nurses supervising nursing students and also the responsibilities of nursing students being supervised by them. This has further drawn out how you need to manage yourself and, to a certain extent, those who support you.

Related to the standards of professional conduct we have briefly considered why nursing is regulated so rigorously by the NMC, primarily respecting their remit to ensure public protection, and again supporting the central role of the patient and the importance of quality care. These discussions should help you to see why expectations of the nursing student to be an accountable professional, committed to lifelong learning, are so important. This chapter has therefore set the foundation that later chapters will build on, in terms of drawing through the individual responsibilities within professional practice. This also sets the scene for consideration of the key transferable skills considered by the NMC to be essential within nursing education.

Activities: Brief outline answers

Activity 1.1 (page 5)

You will all have individual strengths. You have already completed some successful periods of study leading to the qualifications that gained you entry to the nursing course. If you attended a selection event or interview, an experienced nurse has already seen in you the potential to be a nurse. Thinking about your achievements and how you accomplished them may very well enable you to gain insight into what strengths you have.

Activity 1.2 (page 7)

Some ideas include being on time, organised, enthusiastic to do the job and having the skills with which to do so. If you flipped over the role and imagined being the employer, you would want the person to turn up on time and be willing and able to do the job that you were paying them to do. It is often interesting to look at these issues from the other person's perspective.

Activity 1.3 (page 8)

You might have considered that you learn better by doing. That might be what attracted you to the nursing course because you wanted to learn in practice. Think about how you could adapt that in the university. You can be an active learner within the classroom, coming prepared and asking lots of questions. You might also at least in part be a 'theorist', soaking up the knowledge and thinking through what this adds in terms of developing your understanding. Whatever your answer, be prepared to be flexible. Nursing is in many ways defined by its diversity and breadth of underpinning knowledge. You will enjoy the course far more if you make every effort to adapt to each type of learning situation.

Activity 1.4 (page 11)

You might have reflected on how different and individualised your personal choice of dress is from the uniform that you will be wearing as a student. You might not think that you will need to worry about that when you are in the university. But what about when you are in the clinical skills centre practising manual handling or resuscitation? You may well be advised to wear loose casual clothing, flat lace-up shoes and avoid short skirts, as they might prove to be a hindrance in a practical situation. You might be worried if you have a lot of tattoos in highly visible places like your arms or several piercing in your ears or on your face. Some piercings can be removed when in practice or discreetly covered. It would be advisable to check the policies in the Trust where you are placed. Tattoos on your lower arms will clearly not be covered by short-sleeved uniforms, so you may just have to get used to some people asking you about them as they are not easy to remove.

Activity 1.5 (page 11)

With the advent of social networking sites, the landscape of how we can communicate with each other has advanced still further. There are settings you can apply to manage how many people and how much of your personal information is accessible to others. However, care is still needed and you might want to consider your position now. Do you know all of your friends' contacts? It is possible, even if you make your pages only accessible to friends, that other people not known to you might still be able to access your information. There are, of course, guidance notes issued on how to limit or manage your information on these sites, i.e. encouraging you to think about how you can protect yourself. This is important for your personal safety. But some private companies have the capacity to screen sites like Facebook to gain extra insight into the calibre of applicants who apply to work for them. Think about your future. Would you be comfortable for a potential employer to see the information that you post? If you made a derogatory comment about a peer or mentor and this became 'public knowledge' you could find yourself facing a professional suitability review at the university or college where you are studying. The NMC have a high standard of expectation of registrant behaviour, both within and beyond practice. The reality is that you may have to think carefully about the risks of self-disclosure online and through other means.

Activity 1.6 (page 15)

You might have reflected on how vulnerable either you or indeed someone close to you has felt when experiencing a period of illness. Illness can bring with it some unpleasant signs and symptoms. These can include pain, nausea and general malaise. You might have felt worried as to what the diagnosis of the illness was going to be and whether it was serious, which might have been very frightening. When we feel vulnerable, we can quite understandably look to others for advice, information and support. Being in this relatively powerless position of needing some help, it is very important that a comforting and assured response is forthcoming.

You might find it very helpful at regular intervals to consider the position and perspectives of others. This might help you to develop an empathetic response.

Further reading

Cottrell, S (2003) *The Study Skills Handbook*, 2nd edition. Hampshire: Palgrave Macmillan.

This is a popular general guide offering specific advice, activities and illustrations.

Dimond, B (2008) *Legal Aspects of Nursing*, 5th edition. Essex: Longman.

This core text (by a key author within the subject) provides a well written overview of aspects of law pertaining to nursing.

Flynn, R (2004) 'Soft bureacracy', governmentality and clinical governance: theoretical approaches to emergent policy, in Gray, A and Harrison, S (2004) *Governing Medicine, Theory and Practice*. Berkshire: Open University Press.

A demanding read, but nevertheless a book that explains the nature and process of clinical governance in an engaging manner.

Nursing and Midwifery Council (NMC) (2007) *Ensuring Continuity of Practice Assessment Through the Ongoing Achievement Record*. Circular 33. London: NMC.

This issues guidance on maintaining the quality of practice assessment.

Nursing and Midwifery Council (NMC) (2008) *The Code: Standards of conduct, performance and ethics for nurses and midwives*. London: NMC.

Nursing and Midwifery Council (NMC) (2010) *Standards for Pre-registration Nursing Education*. London: NMC.

Both these documents are essential reading for all nursing students.

Sharples, K (2011) *Successful Practice Learning for Nursing Students*. Exeter: Learning Matters.

An essential guide for student nurses on how to prepare for, and get the most out of, practice learning experiences.

Useful websites

http://cqc.org.uk/guidanceforprofessionals/socialcare/careproviders/nationalminimum standards.cfm

The website of the independent regulator of Health and Social Care in England. It lists the Care Quality Commission (2009) National Minimum Standards. It also includes guidance for healthcare professionals and copies of inspection reports.

www.nmc-uk.org

The website of the regulatory body for nurses and midwives, with access to guidance, advice and assistance on individual matters.

Chapter 2
Overview of study and writing skills necessary to be an effective nursing student

Suzanne Waugh

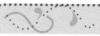 **NMC Standards for Pre-registration Nursing Education**

This chapter will address the following competencies:

Domain 1: Professional values

7. All nurses must be responsible and accountable for keeping their knowledge and skills up to date through continuing professional development. They must aim to improve their performance and enhance the safety and quality of care through evaluation, supervision and appraisal.

9. All nurses must appreciate the value of evidence in practice, be able to understand and appraise research, apply relevant theory and research findings to their work, and identify areas for further investigation.

Domain 4: Leadership, management and team working

3. All nurses must be able to identify priorities and manage time and resources effectively to ensure the quality of care is maintained or enhanced.

4. All nurses must be self-aware and recognise how their own values, principles and assumptions may affect their practice. They must maintain their own personal and professional development, learning from experience, through supervision, feedback, reflection and evaluation.

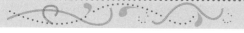 **NMC Essential Skills Clusters**

This chapter will address the following ESCs:

Cluster: Care, compassion and communication

6. People can trust the newly registered graduate nurse to engage therapeutically and actively listen to their needs and concerns, responding using skills that are helpful, providing information that is clear, accurate, meaningful and free from jargon.

continued overleaf . . .

continued . . .

By the first progression point:

1. Communicates effectively both orally and in writing, so that the meaning is always clear.
2. Records information accurately and clearly on the basis of observation and communication.

For entry to the register:

9. Provides accurate and comprehensive written and verbal reports based on the best available evidence.

Cluster: Medicines management

35. People can trust the newly registered graduate nurse to work as part of a team to offer holistic care and a range of treatment options of which medicines may form a part.

For entry to the register:

4. Questions, critically appraises, takes into account ethical considerations and the preferences of the person receiving care and uses evidence to support an argument in determining when medicines may or may not be an appropriate choice of treatment.

Chapter aims

By the end of this chapter, you should be able to:

* manage your time by prioritising your tasks and rearranging your activities to make some more time for yourself;
* understand the purpose of note taking in different settings;
* prepare thoroughly for assignments;
* demonstrate awareness of basic academic writing conventions, such as referencing and writing style;
* analyse sources critically, using questioning;
* identify techniques that will help you perform well in exams;
* appreciate how the study skills you will develop during your course of study will also help you in your nursing career.

Introduction

Beginning your journey as a student nurse might be a daunting prospect. It will probably be very different from any courses you have previously undertaken, with a different structure and ways of learning you may not have encountered before. This chapter takes you through the key study skills you will need in order to successfully complete your course, and gives you tips to help you do well in both your academic studies and career. It will look at how to take good notes, and how to prepare for and produce essays. The chapter will discuss writing skills and critical thinking, and how to avoid plagiarism by referencing correctly. There will also be information about managing your time and preparing for your placements.

Managing your time

As a student nurse, you will find that there are many pressures on your time. You will have classes and placements to attend, along with writing your assignments and all of the preparation needed for them. There will also be many pressures outside of your studies, all competing for your attention – you may have family commitments, possibly a part-time job, not to mention everyday activities such as eating, sleeping, relaxing and socialising to fit into your day. At times, it may all feel a little overwhelming, and you might wonder how you are going to get that essay written on top of attending lectures and looking after your children. It will be hard work – but there are some ways in which you can maximise the time you have available. The key is to prioritise your tasks and to organise your time effectively.

Look at the bigger picture

In order to plan your time, you need to know not just what has to be done right away, but also what is on the horizon. For example, if you have been given three essays to write this semester, you will need to know exactly when each one is due in so that you can plan which one to do first. However, this is not as simple as just saving the key dates in the calendar on your mobile phone – a small screen does not allow you to see the bigger picture. Most people find that using something physically bigger than this will help, so investing in a paper-based diary, calendar or wall planner is money well spent. Many universities and colleges give these away during induction and welcome week, so there is every chance you will be able to get at least one of these items for free.

When you have your diary or planner, add the key dates for your assignments but also for other things that require your time. Being able to see your commitments over several weeks and months at a time will help you to judge how much time you really do have in which you can write your essay. For example, if it is 2 November today, and your essay is due in on 23 November, it might feel like you have plenty of time. However, once you start noting down your other commitments (time on placement – remember that you may have to work antisocial shifts, a weekend away, days when you are in university, social engagements, times when you have personal commitments such as babysitting or driving a friend to an appointment) it becomes apparent that you do not have quite as much time for the essay as it first appeared. It is only by looking at the bigger picture in this way, and working out exactly what tasks you have, that you can begin to plan your time effectively.

Activity 2.1   *Reflection*

Imagine that you are about to complete some coursework for university, and think about the commitments you have for this week. The work will take you at least four hours. Make a list of the things you have to do during the next seven days, and find out how many opportunities there would realistically be for you to complete this assignment.

As this answer is based on your own observation, there is no outline answer at the end of the chapter.

Depending on your other commitments, you may have found it relatively easy or extremely difficult to find time to complete the assignment. The key is to look at the time that you have available in this way, and to prioritise tasks where possible.

Prioritising tasks

There are some tasks that you simply must do – for example, you must not miss your placement or lectures without a good reason, and you cannot push feeding your children to the bottom of your priority list. Therefore, tasks that are both important and urgent must be attended to as a priority. However, there will be other tasks that can be done with a little less urgency, and some that can be moved to another time or ignored completely. When scheduling, consider whether something really is as urgent and/or important as you think it is.

Procrastination

Procrastination is where you put a task off because something else seems far more interesting or exciting. Students often waste time when trying to get started on an essay, for example, because the essay seems like a difficult or unpleasant task, whereas playing a computer game or checking social networking websites seems much more enjoyable. Everyone is guilty of procrastinating sometimes, but if you find yourself doing it frequently, consider the following tips to overcome it.

* Give yourself a reward for doing the task you have been avoiding. For example, if you have been putting off reading a difficult textbook because you find the subject matter hard, reward yourself after 30 minutes of work with 15 minutes of the game/website/other activity of your choice. Having something to look forward to at the end of some hard work will help greatly.
* Think about the consequences of not doing the work you are avoiding. If you fail to complete the report you are meant to be writing, you might fail the module and potentially your course. Remind yourself why you are studying nursing in the first place, and why you want to pass.
* Break the task into more manageable chunks, and tackle an easy part first. Some people find that the opposite helps them, and that doing the most unpleasant part of the task first helps them to complete the rest.
* Ask a friend or family member to check that you have completed the task, and arrange a reward for you both when you have completed it. In this way, you will know that your failure to complete the task will be letting you both down. Sometimes this added pressure helps to spur people on.

Time stealers

As well as procrastinating, we all have activities (or people) who steal our time but which can be rearranged to our advantage.

Activity 2.2   *Reflection*

From your own experience, what could you do differently to give yourself a little more time? Think about things that could be rearranged or changed with relative ease.

As this answer is based on your own experience, there is no outline answer at the end of the chapter. Some examples are discussed below.

Everyone will have a different answer to the question in Activity 2.1, above. However, some suggestions that apply to many people are listed below.

- Watch television at different times. You do not have to stop watching television now that you are a student nurse, but making some small changes to the way in which you watch it can make a big difference. For example, by watching the weekend omnibus of your favourite soap opera instead of watching it every evening, you could free up half an hour each night. This could then be used for digesting the day's study or reading a key text.
- Delegate some tasks. You might be able to ask someone else to do some of the things that take up some of your time. For example, could your partner cook dinner or collect the children sometimes? Every extra half hour will help you to keep on top of your studies.
- Remind other people that your course is important. Sometimes you may have to tell your friend that you will not be able to see him/her until the weekend, because you have to finish your essay.
- Be strict with yourself. If you find that text messages and emails are taking up too much of your time, you might need to leave your mobile phone in another room (or switch it off) while you finish your other tasks. The messages will still be waiting for you when you have finished, but will not be distracting you while you are working.

While studying and when qualified, it is important that you manage your time effectively. As a nurse, you will have many demands on your time and you will need to develop excellent time management skills in order to work effectively. By addressing these issues as a student, you will not only find it easier to meet assignment deadlines, but will also reap the rewards in your future career.

Taking useful notes

As a student nurse, you will need to take good notes in a variety of settings such as lectures, classes and practical sessions. In the library or on the internet, it will be important to make useful notes that will help you with your assignments. While on placement, you may need to note down things you are learning and doing. It is therefore important that you are able to take notes that make sense, cover the important points and help you when you refer back to them at a later date. Note-taking is a skill that many students find difficult at first, but with practice it becomes easier and often eventually becomes second nature. As a qualified nurse, you will be required to keep accurate records, and the writing and note-making skills you develop at university will help you with this.

Taking notes in lectures

When in a lecture or classroom setting, you will need to record the main points that are being discussed. You may be given a handout containing the most important information, in which case you will probably only need to embellish it with explanations and examples. However, if you are not given a handout, the note-taking will be down to you. Remember that you do not need to write down every word, but should be recording the main points. You need to listen to the tutor and understand what they are saying, with your notes acting as a summary of the subjects discussed. Teaching staff are usually happy to clarify or repeat information if you have missed something, such as the spelling of a name or medical terminology, so do not feel afraid to ask the tutor or your fellow students if you did not catch something important.

You will probably find it useful to develop your own shorthand when note-taking, so that you can write more quickly. For example, you might write 'MHN' instead of writing 'mental health nurse' every time. There are some common note-taking shortcuts that many people find useful, such as the small selection shown in Table 2.1.

—	equals (or 'is the same as')
≠	does not equal
♀	female/woman
♂	male/man
∴	because
esp	especially
poss	possibly/possible
ppl	people

Table 2.1: Some common note-taking abbreviations

Taking notes from sources

When reading useful books, journal articles and websites, you will probably want to make some notes to remind you what you have read and what different authors say about a particular topic. Again, the aim is not to copy or reproduce the entire text – rather, you should be summarising what you have read. Try reading a paragraph and then summarising it in a few sentences, or making a list of the most important points. Ideally, you should paraphrase your notes (explain the topic in your own words), but if the author has used a particularly good phrase and you wish to make a note of it, be sure to write the original words in quotation marks in your notes. By doing so, you will know exactly which words were the author's and which were your own. This is very important when using other authors' work in your assignments, which is discussed later in this chapter (see page 32).

Most importantly of all, be sure to record all of the relevant reference details with your notes, so that you can tell exactly which information came from which source. There will be more information about these details later in the chapter (see pages 33–4).

Preparing for assignments

As a higher education student, you will be set several assignments each year that count towards your final qualification. 'Assignment' is a general term that covers many different pieces of work – you may be asked to produce an essay, report, reflective piece of writing or presentation. You may also have to work on a project as a group, which gives you excellent experience for the future, as team work is highly important in nursing.

Assignments help you to understand and digest the topics you have been covering in class or on placement, and allow you to show your tutors that you are progressing well. They also give you the opportunity to look in detail at topics that interest you or are important to your course of study, and practise numerous different skills in order to produce a good piece of work, such as communication skills (written and oral), time management and critical thinking. By communicating clearly with your tutors in assignments, you will be practising the essential skills needed in your career, as you will need to communicate with colleagues and patients. The following tips will help you to prepare for and plan your assignments, so that you can do your best and successfully complete the academic aspects of your training.

Start early

It would be unrealistic to expect every student to begin work on their assignment as soon as the work is set, but it is important that you read the instructions in good time so that you can think about how much work will be involved. You will be able to judge whether the assignment is likely to take a long time and involve a lot of research, or whether it is a shorter assignment for which you already have plenty of information. It is useful to remember that if your entire year group has been set the same assignment, there could potentially be hundreds of students looking for the same books in the library. Preparing yourself in good time should mean that you have plenty of time to access key texts, rather than waiting until the last minute and finding that the library shelves are empty. It is also important to make a note in your diary or on your wall planner or calendar of the submission date of each assignment, so that you can accurately judge how much time you have in which to complete it.

Understand the instructions

You may have been given a question to answer, or a set of instructions detailing how to complete the assignment. Whatever the case, it is important that you understand what you are being asked to produce, the format you should produce it in and any other instructions. First, look at the format required – are you being asked to write an essay (one continuous piece of writing, without headings unless instructed otherwise) or a report (which might contain headings, graphs, charts and have quite a rigid structure)? You must hand in the correct kind of assignment, so be sure to check whether there are any specific instructions about the format of the assignment. Your tutor may, for example, ask you to write a report using particular headings – if you do not follow these instructions, you will lose marks because you will not have done as you were asked.

Next, check the word count for the assignment. Your university or institution will provide you with guidelines as to how many words over or under the word count you are permitted to be – usually, it is either 5 or 10 per cent above or below. For example, if you are asked to write a 2,000 word essay, and your institution allows you to write +/– 10 per cent, you will be allowed to submit essays ranging from 1,800 to 2,200 words. If your essay is outside these boundaries, you will usually lose marks for not following the instructions correctly. Word limits are not there to make the assignment more difficult, they are simply part of your challenge – can you answer this question and discuss all of the important points in a certain amount of words?

If you have been given a choice of questions to answer or are allowed to pick your own topic, choose something that interests you and make sure you feel comfortable with your choice. It is often difficult to motivate yourself when the assignment is not particularly interesting or is very difficult, so if you have a choice of topics, choose carefully and make sure there are enough sources available for your chosen topic.

Now look at the question itself and make sure that you understand what you are being asked to do. If the question is long or complicated, break it into smaller chunks and look at each part in turn. It may help to explain the instructions in your own words, as this will show whether you have understood your task correctly. Try comparing your interpretation of the question to other students' interpretations, and if you do not agree with each other about what you are required to do, check with your tutor. By following the instructions correctly you will not only be increasing your chance of receiving a good mark for your assignment, but you will also be practising skills that will be vital in your placements and professional practice.

Activity 2.3   *Critical thinking*

Look at the following assignment brief. Can you explain what you are being asked to do, in your own words? (Note: Seachester, Rothwell and Hanson have all been invented for the purpose of this chapter.)

Write an essay of 3,000 words, about the following:

Summarise the archaeological evidence from the site at Seachester in Kent, and compare the theories of Rothwell (2009) and Hanson (2010) in relation to these findings.

An outline answer is provided at the end of the chapter.

Start planning your answer

Once you have made sure that you understand what you are being asked to do, it is useful to write a brief plan that summarises this. Your plan will help you to think about the different topics you will need to look up, and to clarify what you already know about the subject. There are no rules about how a plan should look – it is entirely up to you to choose a method that you think will help you. The examples below (Figures 2.1 and 2.2) relate to the question in Activity 2.3 above, and show two different kinds of plan you might find helpful.

These plans look very different, but they both help clarify the question and enable you to direct your research appropriately. Having some initial thoughts and questions in mind before you start

---

- Summarise Seachester's findings (check lecture notes, look up the journal articles mentioned in seminar). Site near the coast, lots of gold jewellery found.
- Rothwell (2009) – look up theory and work.
- Hanson (2010) – discussed in lecture, theory was about ritual burials and evidence of religious worship. Find the journal article mentioned in class.
- Check – has either author written specifically about Seachester?
- Who has written about Seachester? What was their interpretation? Search journal database.

Figure 2.1: Quick essay plan using a list

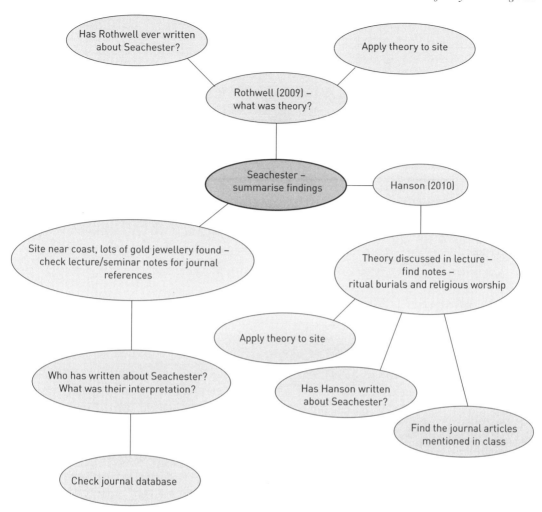

Figure 2.2: Quick essay plan using a spider diagram

reading will be invaluable, as you will have your plan in the back of your mind while you do your research and will be able to look for information in a more targeted way.

Collect the information

Once you know where to start, you will be able to search for the relevant sources more effectively (there is more information on searching for information in Chapter 7). It is good academic practice to use a range of sources, so ideally you need a mixture of books, journal articles, websites or other sources as appropriate. You will probably have been given a reading list by your tutor, and this is a good place to start when looking for relevant information. However, you are expected to find additional material yourself, so you should not rely solely on the sources mentioned by your teachers.

As mentioned above, make sure that you keep a note of the reference for each source used, so that you know where your notes came from.

Update your plan

Before you start writing your answer, it will help if you take some time to update your earlier plan to include what you have found. You may have a lot of information to include, and it is important to think about how you will present this information so that it is clear and easy to understand. You therefore need to plan what you want to say, and the best order in which to say it. Again, this might be in a spider diagram or list, or you might find a flow chart helps. You could even write the various points you wish to make on post-it notes and move them around on the wall, or on a notice board. The way in which you do this is up to you – what matters is that you do some sort of planning before you start writing, so that your essay or report flows in a sensible order and does not jump from one topic to another in a way that is difficult to read.

Remember that your assignment is often the only way you can show your understanding of a certain topic to your tutor. He or she cannot ask you questions about your meaning or argument as they are marking it, so it is very important that they understand what you are writing.

Start writing

If you are finding it difficult to get those first few words written, remember that you do not have to start at the beginning of the essay or report. It might be easier to think about one of the sections you need to include, and start with that. You can always move paragraphs around later if you need to, or change your wording. It is better to get something written than to get stuck because you are not sure how to write the opening line. It is also important to give yourself plenty of breaks while writing, so that you do not become tired and unable to concentrate.

Remember to include a proper introduction, which shows the reader what is going to be discussed in the assignment. You might choose to introduce the topic by defining a key term, or you could open your introduction by explaining what will be covered in the essay or report – for example, 'The purpose of this report is to' . . . Your introduction could be up to 10 per cent of the word count, so it could need to be several hundred words long.

Your conclusion might also be around 10 per cent of the word count, and its purpose is to summarise the points you have been making in the essay or report. You may provide an answer to the original assignment question here, by stating why the evidence has led to a certain conclusion, but you should not discuss any new material at this stage.

It is important to mention that some people find it easiest to write at the computer, whereas others need to write with pen and paper, and then type up the finished assignment. Neither is right or wrong – it is entirely up to you how you get the words on to the page. Do remember, though, that if you write your essay by hand, you will need to set aside enough time to type it up afterwards.

Proofread your draft

When you have written a draft of your assignment, you must spend some time proofreading it. Many people find it difficult to do this using a screen, so if you have done your writing on-screen, it will probably help if you print your work out and read it from paper. You need to check that it makes sense, is easy to follow and does not contain any factual, spelling or grammatical errors.

Although a computer spellchecker can be a helpful tool, it is not a substitute for reading your work through carefully, as a spellchecker cannot understand your intended meaning. Some tips to help you are given below.

Give yourself plenty of time for proofreading

You must allow yourself enough time between completing your draft and proofreading it, so that you have time to digest what you have written properly. Leaving it overnight, or longer if possible, means that the information is not fresh in your mind. You will therefore be able to read your work more objectively, and pick out any weaknesses, rather than reading your work immediately after finishing it and potentially missing errors due to exhaustion. You may also find that additional points that need to be added occur to you during the time between finishing writing and proofreading as your mind processes the information you have been writing about.

Read your assignment out loud

Reading your assignment out loud, either to someone else or just to yourself, will help you to pick up on any grammatical errors or unclear sentences. You or your audience will hear when something is not clear, whereas your eyes might not necessarily pick this up when reading silently. You will notice if you are stumbling over a sentence because of its structure, or if a sentence is particularly long. The clarity of your argument will also be more apparent to your listener when read out loud.

Ask someone else to read it through

It is best to ask someone who is not an expert in the subject or on your course to read the assignment through for you. They may also find that reading it out loud helps, or it may be that a fresh pair of eyes picks up on things that you might not notice yourself. The idea is not that the reader comments on or changes the subject matter, but rather that they comment on the clarity of your argument and the structure of your sentences.

Check that you have answered the original question

When proofreading, bear the assignment instructions or brief in mind and make sure that you have done what you were asked. Ensure that you have not only answered the question and discussed the key themes and theories, but that you have adhered to the word limit and any other instructions given.

Read your feedback

Once your assignment has been marked, you will receive feedback, explaining what you have done well and which areas might need further work. It is important to read this feedback and learn from it, so that you do not repeat mistakes. If you do not understand your tutor's comments, ask for further information – feedback is there to help you and it is important that you take all comments, good or bad, on board.

Basic writing skills

Academic writing is very different from everyday writing such as emailing a friend or writing a letter. You might find it useful to look at some nursing textbooks or journal articles before you begin your studies to get an idea of how academic writing sounds. Writing in this way is excellent practice for your future career, as you will need to keep patient notes and records, or write reports, legally admissible documents or research articles. There are some key points to bear in mind when writing in an academic style.

- You must not use shortened versions (contractions) such as 'don't' or 'can't'. Always use the full version ('do not' or 'cannot').
- Unless you are writing a reflective piece, you will not usually be permitted to use words such as 'I', 'me' or 'we' in your writing. Academic writing almost always uses the third person, so instead of writing 'I don't think this theory is very good', you could write 'It appears that this theory may be flawed, due to' . . . As discussed later, you will need to use other authors' work and the available evidence to back up your claims. However, even without using the word 'I', you will be able to show your own opinions in an academic way, as you will be backing your statements up with evidence and theory.
- You must be particularly careful with your spelling and grammar when writing academic assignments, as you need to show that you are a professional who pays attention to detail and accuracy. By getting into good habits as a student, and checking your writing for these kinds of errors, you will be limiting the likelihood of your making mistakes in your career. It is particularly important to be careful when spelling technical terms and the names of medicines, as inaccuracies could lead to incorrect patient care.

Using another author's work in your assignment

As mentioned above, you will need to back up any claims or opinions in your assignments with evidence. You will do this by referring to the work of other authors and by telling the person reading your assignment what these other authors have said about the topic. Rather than writing about what you think to be the case, you will be looking at every side of the argument and the authors who have written about the topic in order to form a judgement using the available evidence. You will therefore have to think critically about the sources you are using, so that you can compare them and judge their academic value.

Critical thinking

When reading the work of another author, you need to think carefully about what you are reading and ask yourself some questions about the text rather than accepting it at face value. You will therefore need to think in a critical way about the source you read. This does not mean you must be critical in a negative manner, but that you should weigh up the good and bad points of the author's work.

For example, in the example in Activity 2.3, let us suppose Hanson (2010) stated that finding gold jewellery at the site provided undeniable proof of ritual burials. Hanson's opinion was published in a well-respected journal, which usually contains excellent research. However, just because it was published, it is not necessarily true. You would need to look at Hanson's article and find out on what basis this claim was made. What evidence did Hanson present to prove this? Could there be any other interpretations of the items found at the site? Has anyone else written about the subject, and do they agree or disagree with Hanson? By looking more deeply at the sources you read, you will be able to think critically about them and form your own opinions about their validity. You can then discuss their strengths and weaknesses in your assignments, and compare different authors' opinions and arguments.

Activity 2.4   *Critical thinking*

Imagine you are reading an article in a newspaper about student nurses. The article makes the claim that 80 per cent of student nurses dislike working night shifts while on their placements. If you could interview the author about this claim and look at their original research, what questions would you ask in order to find out whether this claim is the truth?

An outline answer is provided at the end of the chapter.

During your career, you will use critical thinking skills regularly. You might need to weigh up the available research in order to make evidence-based choices about patient care, and you may have to explain a patient's choices to them, using the evidence to show potential risks and outcomes. You will therefore need to think critically about the evidence and choices that are available to you, not just as a student nurse, but as a qualified practitioner.

Avoiding plagiarism

When you are writing your essays and reports, you will refer to the work of other authors and discuss what they have said. You must be very careful to say which author's work each piece of information came from so that you do not accidentally plagiarise. Plagiarism means to take the work of another person and pass it off as your own. Therefore, if you find some information in a book by Patel and use this information in your essay without making it clear that it came from Patel's book, you could be accused of plagiarism. It is a very serious academic misconduct offence and the consequences could be severe. It is therefore important that you understand how to avoid plagiarising and are honest in your assignments about whose work you have used.

Referencing

You will need to learn how to reference your work so that you do not accidentally plagiarise. Referencing involves clearly telling the reader where each piece of information has come from by specifying the author(s) whose work you have used. There are many different styles of referencing, or ways it might look on the page, and you will need to check with your tutors which style you are required to learn. However, every style will require you to clearly state whose work you have used and where the information you are discussing has come from. You will usually do this in two places, namely in the body of the essay or report itself and in a reference list at the end of your assignment. It would be impossible to cover every referencing style in this chapter, but the following passage shows an example of how the common Harvard style of referencing might be used in an assignment (the sources are made up for the purpose of this example).

Example

'There have been numerous excavations in the Linden Street area of Seachester in Kent. It is thought by some to have been an army camp in the days before the Battle of Hastings (Smith, 1998; Young, 2001). However, Ryan and Khan (2007) argue that the types of gold jewellery present at the site were not found in northern Europe until at least 1210 AD, some 150 years after the battle of Hastings in 1066. This view has many supporters; most recently Hanson (2010) states that this kind of gold jewellery is only found in England in burial sites dating from the early 1200s onwards. As there is no evidence to suggest human burials at Seachester, this argument has gained more and more supporters in recent years (Hanson, 2010).

Analysis

Alongside each piece of information or academic argument, the original author's name and the year of publication are given to show the reader where the information is from. This can be incorporated into the text (for example, 'Hanson (2010) states...') or can be referenced at the end of the sentence ('...in recent years (Hanson, 2010)').

Note that some information is regarded as common knowledge, and therefore does not require a reference. In this example, the Battle of Hastings is stated to have happened in 1066. There is no debate about this, and it is a known fact. However, if you are writing about an opinion or about something that could be debated, you must always state your source.

To see how the reference list would look using this referencing style, turn to the reference list at the end of this book (pages 214–19).

Exams and assessments

In addition to the written assessments discussed above, you will also have to pass examinations and practical assessments in order to successfully complete your nursing qualification. It is important that you are tested on your knowledge of both theory and practice in order to determine your fitness for practice. A nurse needs to appreciate the reasons for carrying out a procedure in a certain way and the theory behind these actions, as well as being able to carry out the procedure itself.

Academic examinations

Many people find exams stressful, and you may have a negative opinion of them based on your past experience. However, they are a necessary part of university study, and the intention is not to cause stress or anxiety. Exams allow you to show how much of the subject matter you have understood. They are not a simple memory test, but rather a test of your comprehension and ability to apply your knowledge to a certain situation or question. Exams also prepare you for your future career, as nurses frequently need to make decisions or remember procedures under pressure while at work. Rather than seeing exams as frightening, it is useful to put them into perspective and to remember that they are there to help you to consolidate your learning so that you can be a successful practitioner when you qualify.

Some types of exam

The following are some of the kinds of examination you may face at university.

- Multiple choice: you will be given a selection of answers to choose from. If you do not know the answer, you may be able to work out which answer is right by gradually eliminating answers that you know are definitely incorrect. However, as it is possible to score relatively well by merely guessing, multiple choice exams are not used very often in higher education.
- Short answers: there will probably be a large number of questions, all of which require you to write a short paragraph. You will need to revise many topics in order to know a little about everything.
- Essay answers: you will need to write much longer answers (probably several pages long). You will usually only have to answer two or three questions in this kind of exam, so depth of knowledge is essential.
- Oral or presentation: you may have an oral (spoken) examination, where you explain your answers verbally to an examiner. You might also have to give an assessed presentation, in front of an examiner or a panel of tutors. Practising your answers or presentation is vital.

Activity 2.5   *Reflection*

Think about your previous experience of exams and assessment. What kinds of exam have you done before? How did you find them? What do you think you could have done differently?

As this answer is based on your own observation, there is no outline answer at the end of the chapter.

By looking at your own experience, you should be able to identify what has worked well for you in the past, and what has not. The next section of this chapter offers advice that should help you to perform well.

Some tips for written exams

It is important not to leave your revision until the last minute, but rather to start as early as you can. Consolidating the information as you go through the course will help you immensely, so if you have managed to save yourself half an hour a day, as mentioned above, and use this time to go through the day's learning, you will be in an excellent position when it comes to revising. Much of the information will already be stored in your brain and you will understand the topics you have been covering.

Most people find that it works best to revise for short periods of time, with plenty of breaks. Rather than staring at your notes and re-reading everything again and again, try revising actively – can you find any papers from previous years and try to answer the questions while timing yourself? Can you explain a topic out loud? This will show you whether you understand the topic or whether there are things that you need to look up. It can also help to study with someone else and discuss the topics between you. The key is to understand the subject matter and to be able to explain it to someone else in writing – practising doing so verbally or in answer to past paper questions is an excellent way of determining how much you have really understood.

The exam itself can be a stressful situation, but the following tips will help you to perform to your best ability.

- Make sure you know the time and date of the exam, which room it is in (and how to get there), what you can take into the room and how long the exam will last. Get there about 15 minutes before the exam starts, and try to avoid getting involved in panicky conversations about difficult topics.
- When you turn over the exam paper, read it through from start to finish, then read it again. Make sure you know exactly what is expected of you, how many questions to answer (do you have a choice of two from section A, but must answer all from section B?), and start thinking about which questions you could answer first.
- Before you write an essay answer, take some time to plan what you want to say and write a quick plan in your answer booklet. Think about the key points you wish to raise, and also about the structure of your answer. Many students jump straight into answering questions, and end up producing confusing essays that jump between topics as they remember additional information. By planning for a few minutes before you start, you should be able to avoid this, as your answer will already be structured. Examiners like to see essay plans in answer booklets.
- Ignore everyone else. The person next to you might have written a full page before you have even read the paper through, but they have not planned their answers and have probably not even read the question properly. Ignore what everyone else is doing and concentrate on your own answers.
- When you leave the exam, try not to get involved in analysing the paper with other students. Discovering that you answered question four in a completely different way from another student will only cause you to worry about your performance. It is best to just walk away from the exam and wait for your results.

Assessments that test your practical skills

In the last few years, nursing students have increasingly been required to pass a series of objective structured clinical evaluations (OSCEs) as part of their training. These assessments test the student nurse on a variety of competencies, and are your opportunity to show that you not only understand the theory but can apply it to your practice. They involve simulated scenarios in a specially designed laboratory, allowing you to practise techniques such as taking a person's blood pressure in a safe environment without causing harm to 'real' patients. This means that you can develop your skills and improve your performance before entering a 'real' situation (Brosnan et al, 2006). There may also be an oral element to the OSCE, depending on your institution – if so, you will be able to explain verbally why you have made certain decisions. Although you might feel stressed by these practical tests, it is important to remember how useful this practice will be in your future career – evaluations of this new assessment and its impact on students' learning have been overwhelmingly positive (Brosnan et al., 2006; Rentschler et al., 2007; Walsh et al., 2009).

Preparing for your placements

As a student nurse, you will probably spend around half of your course on a clinical placement – the number of weeks spent and the variety of clinical settings will depend on your educational institution. On all placements you will have an allocated mentor who will guide you. You will begin by observing others at work, and will gradually participate more and more in patient care, under the supervision of your mentor. On placement, you will be able to see how the theory you have been learning in class in put into practice in the job itself, and this experience will be invaluable in your development as a practitioner.

In order to get as much as possible out of your placement, you will need to collaborate with your mentor to find opportunities for learning. This means that you will have to be proactive and motivated, seeking out new learning experiences wherever possible, while remembering that your mentor may be busy and at times unable to fully support you (Arkell and Bayliss-Pratt, 2007).

Case study

Tanjia is about to start her next placement. In order to prepare herself as thoroughly as possible, she has done some background research into the kind of institution she will be working at. She has found out who her mentor will be, and plans to get in touch with her mentor beforehand. She is also asking around to find out if any of her fellow students have already attended a placement at the institution. Tanjia is putting a list of questions together which she will ask her mentor or other students, such as what shifts she is likely to be working, where she should park and what the cafeteria is like.

This kind of planning is extremely helpful when getting ready for placements. By finding out as much as possible beforehand, you should feel more confident and be well prepared for the opportunities that await you.

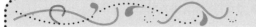

Chapter summary

In this chapter, we have looked at some of the essential study skills that you will need in order to succeed at university. These skills will be important not only for your academic work but also for your placements and career. We have looked at:

- managing your time;
- taking good notes in lectures and from sources;
- planning your assignments;
- basic writing skills;
- using the work of other authors in your assignments;
- preparing for exams and assessments;
- preparing for your placements.

Activities: Brief outline answers

Activity 2.3 (page 28)

Your answer might look something like this:

- I am being asked to write an essay, which will be around 3,000 words long.
- I will need to write a summary of the evidence from Seachester in Kent.
- I must look at Rothwell's theory from 2009.
- I also need to look at Hanson's theory from 2010.
- I then need to see how each theory could be applied to Seachester, and compare them to each other.

Activity 2.4 (page 33)

You could ask the following kinds of question:

(a) How did the author reach this conclusion?
(b) Did they interview student nurses in person, use an online questionnaire etc.?
(c) What questions did they ask? Were they closed 'yes or no' questions, or did individuals have the opportunity to respond as they wished? This is very important, as there is a big difference between Nurse A merely saying 'no' (to a closed question of 'Do you like working nights?') and Nurse B saying 'No, it's not ideal, but it is part of the job to work shifts so I'm perfectly happy to take my turn on nights' (to an open question). Both could be categorised as a 'no' response, but the latter is actually quite positive.
(d) How many student nurses did they ask? Was this a big enough sample size? How were they chosen, and where did the questioning take place?
(e) Did the author remove any findings from the published results?
(f) Looking at the bigger picture, has anyone else done a similar study? What did they find? Do other studies agree or disagree with this research?

Further reading

Burns, T and Sinfield, S (2008) *Essential Study Skills: The complete guide to success at university*, 2nd edition. London: SAGE Publications.

A good general guide to the study skills needed for university, from starting your course to Personal Development Planning.

Cottrell, S (2008) *The Study Skills Handbook*, 3rd edition. Basingstoke: Palgrave Macmillan.

This clearly written book aims to cover all of the basic study skills required for university study.

Hutchfield, K (2010) *Information Skills for Nursing Students*. Exeter: Learning Matters.

A practical and clear guide to mastering information skills, including how to plan and implement a search for information and make judgements on the quality of the sources found.

Sharples, K (2011) *Successful Practice Learning for Nursing Students*. Exeter: Learning Matters.

Useful guidance for student nurses on how to prepare for, and get the most out of, practice learning experiences.

Useful websites

www.careers.salford.ac.uk/studyskills

www.gre.ac.uk/studyskills

There are numerous helpful university study skills websites – try the University of Salford's general guides or the University of Greenwich's pages listed here.

www.nottingham.ac.uk/studentservices/documents/studyskillsfornursesandmidwives.pdf

This is the University of Nottingham's study skills pack aimed specifically at student nurses and midwives.

www.open.ac.uk/skillsforstudy

The Open University's *Skills for OU Study* web pages are an extremely useful resource. Information and advice is given on several study skills topics, such as approaching assignments and exams.

Chapter 3
Being numerate: number skills for nursing practice

Martina O'Brien

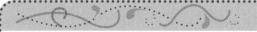

NMC Standards for Pre-registration Nursing Education

This chapter will address the following competencies:

Domain 1: Professional values

8. All nurses must practise independently, recognising the limits of their competence and knowledge. They must reflect on these limits and seek advice from, or refer to, other professionals where necessary.

Domain 3: Nursing practice and decision-making

5. All nurses must understand public health principles, priorities and practice in order to recognise and respond to the major causes and social determinants of health, illness and health inequalities. They must use a range of information and data to assess the needs of people, groups, communities and populations, and work to improve health, wellbeing and experiences of healthcare; secure equal access to health screening, health promotion and healthcare; and promote social inclusion.

6. All nurses must practise safely by being aware of the correct use, limitations and hazards of common interventions, including nursing activities, treatments, and the use of medical devices and equipment. The nurse must be able to evaluate their use, report any concerns promptly through appropriate channels and modify care where necessary to maintain safety. They must contribute to the collection of local and national data and formulation of policy on risks, hazards and adverse outcomes.

NMC Essential Skills Clusters

This chapter will address the following ESCs:

Cluster: Organisational aspects of care

9. People can trust the newly registered graduate nurse to treat them as partners and work with them to make a holistic and systematic assessment of their needs; to develop a

continued opposite . . .

continued . . .

personalised plan that is based on mutual understanding and respect for their individual situation promoting health and well-being, minimising risk of harm and promoting their safety at all times.

By the second progression point:

2. Accurately undertakes and records a baseline assessment of weight, height, temperature, pulse, respiration and blood pressure using manual and electronic devices.

6. Measures and documents vital signs under supervision and responds appropriately to findings outside the normal range.

8. Collects and interprets routine data, under supervision, related to the assessment and planning of care from a variety of sources.

Cluster: Nutrition and fluid management

27. People can trust the newly registered graduate nurse to assist them to choose a diet that provides an adequate nutritional and fluid intake.

By the second progression point:

2. Accurately monitors dietary and fluid intake and completes relevant documentation.

28. People can trust the newly registered graduate nurse to assess and monitor their nutritional status and in partnership, formulate an effective plan of care.

By the second progression point:

1. Takes and records accurate measurements of weight, height, length, body mass index and other appropriate measures of nutritional status.

29. People can trust a newly registered graduate nurse to assess and monitor their fluid status and in partnership with them, formulate an effective plan of care.

By the second progression point:

2. Accurately monitors and records fluid intake and output.

3. Recognises and reports reasons for poor fluid intake and output.

Cluster: Medicines management

33. People can trust the newly registered graduate nurse to correctly and safely undertake medicines calculations.

By the first progression point:

1. Is competent in basic medicines calculation relating to:
   - tablets and capsules
   - liquid medicines
   - injections including:
     - unit dose
     - sub and multiple unit dose
     - SI unit conversion

> **Chapter aims**
>
> By the end of this chapter, you should be able to:
>
> - understand the mathematical principles that underpin the safe delivery of nursing care;
> - demonstrate the ability to perform accurate numeracy calculations in a wide range of nursing care activities;
> - identify the relevance of numerical data to nursing care interventions.

Introduction

Being numerate is a fundamental principle that underpins the safe delivery of a wide range of nursing care activities. This chapter explores the various numerical skills that are required by the Nursing and Midwifery Council (NMC) to enable you to provide safe and effective care to your patients. Being numerate should enable you not only to recognise and administer the correct doses of medicines, but also allow you to understand the hydration and nutritional status of your patients. It will allow you to understand their physiological observations and interpret a variety of assessments used in patient care. Understanding the numerical data will enable you to intervene, report and deliver the most appropriate care to your patients. Areas to be covered in this chapter include basic calculation skills, fluid balance and nutritional status, interpreting patient data such as graphs, charts and vital signs, calculating medicine doses and intravenous infusion rates and interpreting specimen results.

Basic calculation skills

This section will enable you to check your understanding of basic mathematical principles. If you are not already familiar with how to add, subtract, multiply or divide, you should review these principles before you continue reading this chapter. It is also worthwhile refreshing your understanding of how to deal with fractions, decimals, percentages and ratios. A useful book to read is *Passing Calculations Tests for Nursing Students* (Starkings and Krause, 2010). By working through a variety of mathematical exercises, you should be able to self-assess your abilities with all of the above. Completing these activities will help you achieve the necessary proficiency for entry into your field of practice programme.

Answer the questions related to the following scenarios to see if you understand the principles of addition and subtraction.

> **Activity 3.1**
>
> A learning disabilities unit is comprised of two day centres, a short-stay residential floor and a community school. The day centres have the capacity to cater for 15 and 21 young
>
> *continued opposite . . .*

continued . . . •

adults respectively. The short-stay residential floor offers respite care to teenagers and is able to accommodate a maximum of 11 residents at any one time. The community school has two classrooms each able to cater for 14 teenagers in each room.

(a) How many young adults and teenagers can be accommodated in the unit at any given time?

(b) On Monday last week the day centres catered for a total of 19 young adults and the community school taught 21 teenagers. The residential floor had two residents. How many more people could the unit have catered for?

(c) The residential floor and one of the classrooms is temporarily closing due to financial constraints. How many fewer teenagers will be able to attend the unit as a result of these cost-cutting measures?

The Ward Manager has been allocated £32,000 to spend on training courses and study days for her staff for the forthcoming year. Staff Nurse Halls is about to commence studies on a palliative care course at the local university at a cost of £800. Junior Sister Waterhouse has been granted funding for the second year of her Masters programme of study at a cost of £4,500. An additional four members of staff will be commencing their mentorship preparation courses at a cost of £900 per person. Two Health Care Assistants (HCAs) have been granted permission to attend a half-day conference on clinical skills at a cost of £125 per person.

(d) How much of the initial £32,000 is remaining after all the courses and study days have been paid for?

(e) One of the HCAs realises that the conference she has booked onto clashes with a holiday she has already booked. What is the total spend now for all the courses and study days?

The correct answers are provided at the end of the chapter.

Now try the following calculations to test your understanding of the principles of multiplication and division.

Activity 3.2

(a) 32 × 36   (d) 96 ÷ 3
(b) 452 × 5   (e) 1001 ÷ 11
(c) 232 × 4

The correct answers are provided at the end of the chapter.

Using calculators

We use many basic mathematical principles in our daily lives in tasks ranging from working out our utility bills and paying for our groceries to working out the interest rates on our savings or credit card. Many of us use calculators to perform such tasks. However, it is important to remember that the answers delivered by a calculator can only be as accurate as the information put into it by the user. More often than not it is human error that results in mistakes being made. In order to input correct information you still need to understand the basics of maths. When using calculators to work out a mathematical calculation, it is vital that the correct information is put into the calculator and in the correct format. Depending on the calculator you use, it may be necessary to subtotal calculations where more than two sets of numbers are involved.

For example: $9 + 6 \times 3$

Inputting the numbers and the mathematical signs like that will provide an answer of 27 on some calculators, which is wrong. The correct answer is 45. To ensure you accurately calculate this sum it is necessary to input the information in two stages, as follows:

$9 + 6 = 15 \times 3 = 45$

The NMC offers guidance on the use of calculators. They advise for complex drug calculations *that it is good practice for a second practitioner (a registered professional) to check the calculation independently in order to minimise the risk of error. The use of calculators to determine the volume or quantity of medication should not act as a substitute for arithmetical knowledge and skill* (NMC, 2007, p38).

Fractions

While fractions are not used as much as whole numbers or decimals, you still need to know how to work with them. For example, there will be occasions when, as a nursing student, you will be expected to administer part of an ampoule of medication or part of a tablet. Try the following exercise to test your understanding of how to add and subtract fractions (remember to convert to equivalent fractions when needed and to simplify fractions where possible).

Activity 3.3

(a) $\dfrac{3}{5} + \dfrac{2}{3}$

(b) $\dfrac{4}{8} + \dfrac{3}{4}$

(c) $\dfrac{3}{8} - \dfrac{1}{10}$

(d) $\dfrac{1}{5} + \dfrac{2}{3} - \dfrac{1}{3}$

(e) $\dfrac{1}{3} - \dfrac{1}{12} + \dfrac{4}{18} + \dfrac{1}{3}$

The correct answers are provided at the end of the chapter.

Now try the following exercise to test your understanding of how to multiply and divide fractions.

Activity 3.4

(a) $\dfrac{2}{8} \times \dfrac{1}{2}$

(b) $\dfrac{1}{3} \times \dfrac{1}{3}$

(c) $\dfrac{2}{3} \div \dfrac{1}{4}$

(d) $\dfrac{4}{9} \div \dfrac{1}{6}$

(e) $\dfrac{1}{3} \times \dfrac{1}{8} \div \dfrac{3}{9}$

The correct answers are provided at the end of the chapter.

Decimals

Fractions or parts of a whole number can also be expressed as decimal numbers. Nurses use decimals on a regular basis – for example, during medicine administration or when calculating the weight of a patient. Try the following exercise to test your understanding of adding, subtracting, multiplying and dividing decimals. Remember to round off any numbers after the decimal point.

Activity 3.5

Where possible give answers to two decimal places.

(a) $0.02 + 0.03$

(b) $12.87 - 11.23$

(c) 23.6×2.4

(d) $1.9 \div 0.3$

(e) $0.002 \times 0.03 \div 0.07$

The correct answers are provided at the end of the chapter.

Converting fractions to decimals and decimals to fractions

It is more usual to convert fractions to decimals rather than the other way round, because in nursing we tend to use the metric system when dealing with numbers.

Electronic devices such as pumps used to administer medicine dosages to patients have metric calibrations, which need to be programmed to run at set rates of infusion. This might involve the nurse inputting whole and decimal numbers to ensure the pump runs at the correct rate to give the patient the correct medicine dosage. Medicines in general are prescribed in decimals rather than fractions. Medicine dosages will be covered later in this chapter (see pages 63–6).

Activity 3.6

Convert the following fractions to decimals. Round off to two decimal places where possible.

(a) $\dfrac{2}{4}$

(b) $\dfrac{1}{3}$

(c) $\dfrac{4}{9}$

Convert the following decimals to fractions:

(d) 0.25

(e) 0.5

The correct answers are provided at the end of the chapter.

Percentages

Per cent means 'part of a hundred' or 'out of a hundred'. For example, 40 per cent means 40 out of 100. Percentages are useful as they can give significance to a number. For example, if it was known that 97 per cent of patients suffered side effects of a new medicine, this would indicate that most people had undesirable effects from the medicine (97 out of 100 people). It would probably be wise to consider asking the doctor to prescribe an alternative medication.

Percentages are also useful when making comparisons. So if, for example, 97 per cent of patients suffered side effects with a new medicine and 2 per cent of patients suffered similar effects with an alternative medicine, it would seem prudent for the alternative medicine to be the one of choice.

In nursing you will come across many examples of where percentages are used. For example, the components of a medicine may be expressed as 0.9 per cent sodium chloride, 50 per cent glucose and so on. During your studies you will read many research articles where the results of studies are given in percentages.

Try the following exercise to test your understanding of percentages.

Activity 3.7

Round off your answers to the nearest whole number.

(a) 10% of 300

(b) 42% of 83

continued opposite . . .

continued . . .

Now express the following values as a percentage (again round off answers to the nearest whole percentage point).

(c) 49 out of 98
(d) 865 out of 870
(e) 3 out of 14

The correct answers are provided at the end of the chapter.

Ratios

Ratios are used when you want to compare the relationship of one quantity to another. So, for example, if you read a research study that indicated a ratio of 1:3 people took part in the study, then this would tell you that for every person who participated in the study, three did not. In other words, for every four people that may have been approached to take part in it, only one person did so. This may help you to decide whether the study and its findings are credible and perhaps can be generalised to a population of people. There are numerous situations where ratios are used. For example, during your learning opportunity placements you will discover ratios being used to determine how many registered nurses are needed to work a span of duty. Your university will probably use ratios when determining how many nursing lecturers it needs to employ to teach the number of nursing students on your course.

Take a look at the following example.

Worked example

Martina and Joan raised a total of £1600 during a fundraising raffle, in the ratio of 5:3. How much money did each person raise?

To work this out you need to determine how many 'shares' there are.

So 5 + 3 = 8 shares.

continued overleaf . . .

Next, you need to work out how much one share is worth. Simply divide £1600 by 8.

So 1600 ÷ 8 = 200.

In other words one share is equal to £200.

Since Martina raised 5 shares you need to multiply £200 x 5 = £1000.

Joan raised 3 shares, so £200 x 3 = £600.

Therefore in this example the ratio 5:3 tells you that Martina raised £1000 for the raffle while Joan raised £600.

Try the following exercise to test your understanding of ratios.

Activity 3.8

(a) In total, between them, Hannah and James have accumulated 24 years of nursing experience, in a ratio of 1:5. How many years' experience has each accumulated?

(b) In the learning disabilities unit, the ratio of registered nurses to Health Care Assistants is 3:2. If there are 24 registered nurses, how many Health Care Assistants are employed on the unit?

(c) The pass rate for an exam for the last 3 cohorts of nursing students is expressed in the following ratio: 5:4:3. A total of 360 students passed the exam. How many were successful in each cohort?

The correct answers are provided at the end of the chapter.

Maintaining proficiency in numerical calculations

You may find that your ability to perform numerical calculations lessens over time. As with any skill it is important to practise to maintain your proficiency.

This section has enabled you to understand the basic mathematical principles that you will need to use in the safe delivery of nursing care. The following sections of this chapter will focus on specific areas of care where numeracy skills are required. If you have found any difficulty in the activities, then you need to revise your basic arithmetic until you are confident in your understanding, accuracy and speed. The BBC Bitesize and the HEA Mathcentre online resources offer revision material that you can access to improve your skills. Website addresses can be found at the end of this chapter.

Understanding fluid balance and nutritional status

This section will enable you to accurately calculate the hydration and nutritional status of your patients. You will become familiar with how to assess a patient's nutritional status to determine whether they are malnourished. The prompt detection of dehydrated or fluid overloaded patients and the importance of the accurate completion of fluid balance charts will also be explored.

Fluid balance

There are many factors that affect how fluids and **electrolytes** are used and maintained in the body: age, exercise, diet and health status are just some of these factors. In a healthy individual the body is able to maintain a balance between the fluid that it takes in and the fluid it excretes, or loses. In simple terms this means that in a 24-hour period a healthy individual should excrete about the same amount of fluid that he or she has taken in. If fluid intake is more than what is excreted, the patient is said to be in a **positive fluid balance** as the body has retained fluid. Conversely, if more fluid is excreted than is taken in, the patient is in a **negative fluid balance** since the body has lost fluid.

Patients' fluid intake and output are recorded on a fluid balance chart similar to the one in Figure 3.1. It is used to assess the hydration status of patients. It is important that you understand how to complete and interpret the charts as the care and treatment you give your patients will be determined by the information on the chart and your interpretation of it.

The 24-hour clock is used on charts so as to avoid any confusion between morning, afternoon, evening and night times. So, for example, 06.00 on a chart means that the time referred to is 6 o'clock in the morning and 18.00 is 6 o'clock in the evening.

VALLEY HILLS NHS FOUNDATION TRUST

PATIENT NAME:	HOSPITAL NUMBER:	DATE OF BIRTH:	WARD:	CONSULTANT:

DATE:

		INPUT			OUTPUT		
TIME	ORAL	I.V	I.V	URINE	VOMIT/NG	DRAIN
01.00						
02.00						
03.00						
04.00						
05.00						
06.00						
07.00						
08.00						
09.00						
10.00						
11.00						
12.00						
13.00						
14.00						
15.00						
16.00						
17.00						
18.00						
19.00						
20.00						
21.00						
22.00						
23.00						
24.00						
TOTALS						
TOTAL INPUT/OUTPUT						
FLUID BALANCE POSITIVE/NEGATIVE						

Figure 3.1: Fluid balance chart

Nutritional status

Patients should have their nutritional status assessed and recorded when they are admitted to hospital. This should be regularly reassessed, particularly if or when there are changes in their condition. For some patients you will need to record any food or fluids that they consume that have nutritional value. This is needed so that it can be determined how many calories they are taking in and whether that amount is too much or too little to meet their body's nutritional requirements. Understanding the nutritional status of your patients will enable you to understand laboratory test results, which will be covered later in this chapter (see pages 69–70).

A nutritional risk assessment is carried out to ascertain whether the patient is malnourished. A popular tool used in adult nursing is the Malnutrition Universal Screening Tool (MUST) developed by the Malnutrition Advisory Group (BAPEN, 2003). You can download the tool from **www.bapen.org.uk/pdfs/must/must_full.pdf**. It requires a variety of data to be collected from your patient, culminating in a numerical score to determine their risk of malnutrition.

- 0 = low risk
- 1 = medium risk
- 2 or more = high risk

Care is then planned to address the risk of malnutrition.

Activity 3.9

Read the following scenario and complete the fluid balance chart in Figure 3.1.

Benji Todd is a six-year-old boy admitted to Oak Ward with renal failure. He has a urinary catheter and an intravenous infusion (IVI) *in situ*. Part of his treatment requires strict fluid balance monitoring. You are required to complete the fluid balance chart in Figure 3.1 as a record of his fluid input and output for the last 24 hours. Other data you require is as follows:

- Date of birth: 12/12/2004
- Hospital number: 120967
- Consultant: Mr Roberts

Benji drank half a beaker of water at 06.00 to help him swallow his medicine. His urinary catheter was emptied at 07.00; it contained 525ml of urine. He consumed a cup of warm milk at 09.00 and had half a beaker of milk poured onto his breakfast cereal, and he ate all of it. His IVI of 500ml commenced at 03.00 and ran at a rate of 50ml per hour. He had no more IVI fluids after this one had completed. At 10.00 he drank two-thirds of a beaker of orange squash. At 12.00 and 15.00 he drank a beaker of water. For lunch at 13.00 he consumed half a bowl of tomato soup. At 18.00 he drank a strawberry milkshake (a beaker full). Unfortunately, Benji vomited 100ml of fluid shortly after consuming the milkshake. Before he went to bed at 20.00 he had a cup of hot chocolate. At midnight his urinary catheter was emptied of 650 ml of urine.

To assist you with this activity please use the following measurements.

- A beaker holds 150ml.
- A cup holds 125ml.
- A bowl holds 300ml.

(a) What is the total fluid input and output for Benji during this 24-hour period?
(b) Is his fluid balance positive or negative and by how much?

An outline answer of what you may have considered is provided at the end of this chapter, including a completed copy of the fluid balance chart.

This section has enabled you to accurately document and interpret data related to patients' hydration and nutrition status. The next section will look at further charts that you will be expected to use during your practice learning opportunities.

Interpreting graphs and charts

You can learn a lot about your patient's health from numerical data recorded on graphs and charts. Such data can provide you with a useful overview of the progress your patient is making. It can also alert you to any deterioration in your patient's condition, which will enable you to intervene and take the necessary action to improve matters. This section will explore the use of some of the graphs and charts that you may use in patient care.

When patients attend for any form of healthcare, be it at an outpatients clinic, a walk-in centre or as a hospital inpatient, they will invariably undergo various forms of assessment in order to obtain data that can assist the healthcare professional in understanding their health status. Consider the following scenario.

> ### Case study
>
> *Ian is a 43-year-old man who regularly attends the obesity clinic at his local NHS Trust. He is one of the 24 per cent of men found to be obese in the UK (The Health and Social Care Information Centre, 2010). He is on a dietary and exercise regimen in an effort to reduce his weight. At his most recent appointment Ian was found to have BMI of 31 (kg/m²) and a waist circumference of 104cm; both these measurements means he is classified as obese.*

Body Mass Index (BMI)

Obesity can be measured in a variety of ways. For example, weighing somebody will allow you to compare their weight with the average weight of someone who is of similar height and build (and age in the case of children). The most common way to determine whether someone is overweight or obese is to calculate their Body Mass Index (BMI). This is calculated by dividing the patient's weight (in kilograms) with their height (in metres squared). A quicker and simpler method of doing this is to use a BMI chart, like the one in Figure 3.2

> ### Activity 3.10
>
> Calculate your BMI using the formula described in the section above. You can confirm whether your calculations are correct by using a BMI chart, like the one in Figure 3.2.
>
> *As this exercise is dependent on individual measurements, there is no outline answer provided.*

Body Mass Index (BMI) Chart for Adults

Obese (>30) Overweight (25-30) Normal (18.5-25) Underweight (<18.5)

HEIGHT in feet/inches and centimeters

WEIGHT		4'8"	4'9"	4'10"	4'11"	5'0"	5'1"	5'2"	5'3"	5'4"	5'5"	5'6"	5'7"	5'8"	5'9"	5'10"	5'11"	6'0"	6'1"	6'2"	6'3"	6'4"	6'5"
lbs	(kg)	142cm	147	150	152	155	157	160	163	165	168	170	173	175	178	180	183	185	188	191	193	196	
260	(117.9)	58	56	54	53	51	49	48	46	45	43	42	41	40	38	37	36	35	34	33	32	32	31
255	(115.7)	57	55	53	51	50	48	47	45	44	42	41	40	39	38	37	36	35	34	33	32	31	30
250	(113.4)	56	54	52	50	49	47	46	44	43	42	40	39	38	37	36	35	34	33	32	31	30	30
245	(111.1)	55	53	51	49	48	46	45	43	42	41	40	38	37	36	35	34	33	32	31	31	30	29
240	(108.9)	54	52	50	48	47	45	44	43	41	40	39	38	36	35	34	33	33	32	31	30	29	28
235	(106.6)	53	51	49	47	46	44	43	42	40	39	38	37	36	35	34	33	32	31	30	29	29	28
230	(104.3)	52	50	48	46	45	43	42	41	39	38	37	36	35	34	33	32	31	30	30	29	28	27
225	(102.1)	50	49	47	45	44	43	41	40	39	37	36	35	34	33	32	31	31	30	29	28	27	27
220	(99.8)	49	48	46	44	43	42	40	39	38	37	36	34	33	32	32	31	30	29	28	27	27	26
215	(97.5)	48	47	45	43	42	41	39	38	37	36	35	34	33	32	31	30	29	28	28	27	26	25
210	(95.3)	47	45	44	42	41	40	38	37	36	35	34	33	32	31	30	29	28	28	27	26	26	25
205	(93.0)	46	44	43	41	40	39	37	36	35	34	33	32	31	30	29	29	28	27	26	26	25	24
200	(90.7)	45	43	42	40	39	38	37	35	34	33	32	31	30	30	29	28	27	26	26	25	24	24
195	(88.5)	44	42	41	39	38	37	36	35	33	32	31	31	30	29	28	27	26	26	25	24	24	23
190	(86.2)	43	41	40	38	37	36	35	34	33	32	31	30	29	28	27	26	26	25	24	24	23	23
185	(83.9)	41	40	39	37	36	35	34	33	32	31	30	29	28	27	27	26	25	24	24	23	23	22
180	(81.6)	40	39	38	36	35	34	33	32	31	30	29	28	27	27	26	25	24	24	23	22	22	21
175	(79.4)	39	38	37	35	34	33	32	31	30	29	28	27	27	26	25	24	24	23	22	22	21	21
170	(77.1)	38	37	36	34	33	32	31	30	29	28	27	27	26	25	24	24	23	22	22	21	21	20
165	(74.8)	37	36	34	33	32	31	30	29	28	27	26	25	24	24	23	22	22	21	21	20	20	
160	(72.6)	36	35	33	32	31	30	29	28	27	27	26	25	24	24	23	22	22	21	21	20	19	19
155	(70.3)	35	34	32	31	30	29	28	27	27	26	25	24	24	23	22	22	21	20	20	19	19	18
150	(68.0)	34	32	31	30	29	28	27	27	26	25	24	23	23	22	22	21	20	20	19	19	18	18
145	(65.8)	33	31	30	29	28	27	27	26	25	24	23	22	22	21	21	20	20	19	19	18	18	17
140	(63.5)	31	30	29	28	27	26	26	25	24	23	23	22	21	21	20	20	19	18	18	17	17	17
135	(61.2)	30	29	28	27	26	26	25	24	23	22	22	21	21	20	19	19	18	18	17	17	16	16
130	(59.0)	29	28	27	26	25	25	24	23	22	22	21	20	20	19	19	18	18	17	17	16	16	15
125	(56.7)	28	27	26	25	24	24	23	22	21	21	20	19	18	18	17	17	16	16	16	15	15	15
120	(54.4)	27	26	25	24	23	23	22	21	21	20	19	19	18	18	17	17	16	16	15	15	15	14
115	(52.2)	26	25	24	23	22	22	21	20	20	19	19	18	17	17	16	16	16	15	15	14	14	14
110	(49.9)	25	24	23	22	21	21	20	19	19	18	18	17	17	16	16	15	15	15	14	14	13	13
105	(47.6)	24	23	22	21	21	20	19	19	18	17	17	16	16	15	15	14	14	13	13	13	13	12
100	(45.4)	22	22	21	20	20	19	18	18	17	17	16	16	15	15	14	14	14	13	13	13	12	12
95	(43.1)	21	21	20	19	19	18	17	17	16	16	15	15	14	14	14	13	13	13	12	12	12	11
90	(40.8)	20	19	19	18	18	17	16	16	15	15	15	14	14	13	13	13	12	12	12	11	11	11
85	(38.6)	19	18	18	17	17	16	16	15	15	14	14	13	13	12	12	12	11	11	11	11	10	10
80	(36.3)	18	17	17	16	16	15	15	14	14	13	13	13	12	12	11	11	11	11	10	10	10	9

Note: BMI values rounded to the nearest whole number. BMI categories based on CDC (Centers for Disease Control and Prevention) criteria.
www.vertex42.com   BMI = Weight[kg] / (Height[m] x Height[m]) = 703 x Weight[lb] / (Height[in] x Height[in])   © 2009 Vertex42 LLC

Figure 3.2: Body Mass Index chart

Charts can also be used to plot your patient's weight, for example. Using several measurements you can tell if the patient loses, gains or remains a steady weight. Weight measurements are needed for a variety of reasons. They can be used as an indicator of how efficiently the heart is working, to monitor progress on a calorie controlled dietary intake, to calculate a patient's BMI (as discussed above), to calculate how much of a medicine to give a patient and so on.

Centile charts

Charts are used for babies and children to check if they have a healthy pattern of growth. Growth is an important measure of how healthy a child is. The expected pattern of growth is based on data from babies who have been breastfed in optimal conditions in six different countries (Royal College of Paediatrics and Child Health, 2009). At key stages of a baby or child's development, the weight, height (or length depending on the age of the child) and head circumference are measured and plotted on the growth chart. These measurements are plotted on centile lines. Each centile marks the percentage at which an individual of the same age and gender falls. So, for example, if a child's height is marked at the 25th centile this means that they are one of the 25 per cent of children in their age group and gender who are of similar height. In essence, this would mean that they are shorter in height than the average child of their age and gender. You can access the various charts used at **www.rcpch.ac.uk/Research/UK-WHO-Growth-Charts**.

This section has looked at some charts and graphs that you will need to use during your learning opportunities to assist in determining the health status of your patients. The next section will address the importance of risk assessments in patient care.

Risk assessments

It is much better to identify a risk to a patient than allow them to be exposed to harm. This section will discuss the use of some numerical risk assessment tools that are used in practice to identify the risk of harm to your patients. Risk assessment tools are designed to assist the nurse in understanding the likelihood of a patient being at risk of, for example, developing pressure ulcers or being or becoming malnourished. Care and interventions can then be planned in light of these assessment results to reduce or prevent a risk.

Activity 3.11

List the types of numerical assessments you have seen being used during your learning opportunities to determine a risk to your patients.

An outline answer is provided at the end of the chapter.

Pressure ulcer risk assessment tools

You may have considered the MUST tool that was discussed earlier in this chapter (see page 51) to assess a patient's risk of malnutrition. Another very important aspect of patient care is that of identifying those patients who have **pressure ulcers** or are at risk of developing them. Pressure ulcers, previously called pressure sores, affect the skin and underlying tissue, usually over a bony prominence such as the heel of the foot, elbows, sacrum, and so on. They are caused by unrelieved pressure on that area, for example sitting in a chair for too long without moving. They can also be caused by pressure combined with a shearing or friction force – for example, a patient being dragged up the bed without the use of appropriate moving and handling equipment such as **sliding sheets**. There are many other factors that place a patient at risk of developing them. In order to identify those at risk your Hospital Trust will use a risk assessment tool. You may find that different wards and departments within the same Hospital Trust use different ones. This is because there are so many tools available, some of which are better suited to one area than to another.

Here are just some of the tools that you may use.

- The Waterlow Scale, which identifies those who are 'at risk', 'high risk' and 'very high risk' after a series of patient data is collected (Waterlow, 1985).

- The Norton Score, which requires collection of patient data, each given a numerical score. A score under 14 indicates that a patient is at risk of developing a pressure ulcer (Norton et al., 1975).
- Pressure Sore Prediction Score (PSPS), which is primarily for orthopaedic patients and consists of six questions with required answers to be either 'yes', 'yes, but', 'no' or 'no, but'. Each answer has a numerical value assigned to it. A score of six or above indicates a patient is at risk of developing a pressure ulcer (Lowthian, 1987).

Those patients who are assessed as being at high risk of pressure ulcer development should then have their care planned in a manner that reduces this risk. Care interventions may include regular assistance with changing position and using special bed mattresses or seat cushions that help to relieve pressure.

As you have learnt from this section, while basic numerical skills are needed to complete accurate risk assessments, you also need clinical expertise to implement appropriate care to reduce risks for your patients.

Interpreting vital signs

The accurate monitoring and interpreting of vital signs is an important nursing procedure that you will be expected to carry out many times on each shift of every learning opportunity placement. This section will cover the normal parameters and units of measurement to look for when performing checks on your patient's vital signs. Blood pressure (BP), temperature (T), pulse (P) and respiratory rates (R), and oxygen saturations (SpO_2) will be explored. The importance of these vital signs and their relationship to treating critically ill patients will also be explored by the use of Early Warning Scores (EWS).

When patients first come into a healthcare setting they should always have their vital signs taken and documented on an observation chart similar to the one in Figure 3.3 below. These readings will act as a baseline. As your patient undergoes treatment you will be expected to monitor their vital signs at regular intervals to determine how they are responding to any care intervention. Then, as their care and treatment progresses, you will quickly be able to determine whether there are any marked deviations from their baseline readings. If there is, this may indicate that there is deterioration in their condition. Your understanding of any such changes, any action you take and how quickly you respond as a result of your interpretation of these changes will very much influence how your patient recovers and whether they will need any further treatments.

The chart in Figure 3.3 has recorded the vital signs of Jonas Devises for a span of three days. Each square box on the chart is divided into units of ten (for blood pressure, pulse and respiration recordings) and tenths (for temperature recordings). You can see that there are some fluctuations in the readings. To determine whether Mr Devises' vital signs are within normal limits you need to know what the parameter ranges are for each vital sign.

Table 3.1 lists the most common vital signs that are measured with the normal parameters for children and adults. It is important to note that there are several factors that will impact on your patient's vital signs, such as age, environment, level of physical activity, metabolic rate, time of day, medication, infection, menstrual cycle, eating, disease, posture, gravity, emotional factors and **'white coat syndrome'** (Maddex, 2009).

VALLEY HILLS NHS FOUNDATION TRUST

PATIENT NAME:	HOSPITAL NUMBER:	DATE OF BIRTH:	WARD:	CONSULTANT:
Jonas Devises	386534	31/10/39	Delta	Mr Hills

	1st November 2010						2nd November 2010						3rd November 2010					
	02.00	06.00	10.00	14.00	18.00	22.00	02.00	06.00	10.00	14.00	18.00	22.00	02.00	06.00	10.00	14.00	18.00	22.00
40°C																		
39°C																		
38°C	■																	
37°C		■		■	■							■						
36°C			■			■			■						■			
35°C																		
170																		
160																		
150																		
140			V			V									V			
130			I	V	V	I						V			I			
120	V	V	I	I	I	I			V						I			
110	I	I	I	I	I	I			I						I			
100	I	I	I	I	I	I			I						I			
90	I	I	^	I	I	^			I			I			^			
80	I	I		^	^	X			I			^			X			
70	^	^	X	X					^									
60	X	X			X				X			X						
50																		
40																		
30																		
20	■	■	■						■									
10				■		■						■			■			
0																		

Figure 3.3: Observation chart

Vital sign	Unit of measurement	Normal parameters: children	Normal parameters: adult
Temperature (T)	Celsius °C	36°C–37°C	36°C–37.4°C
Blood pressure (BP)	Millimetres of mercury: mmHg	Systolic: 95–115mmHg Diastolic: 55–70mmHg (age dependent)	Systolic: 100–140mmHg Diastolic: 60–90mmHg
Pulse (P)	Beats per minute (bpm)	Newborn: 100–180 bpm Infant: 110–160 bpm 1–2 yrs: 100–150 bpm 2–5 yrs: 95–140 bpm 5–12 yrs: 80–120 bpm Adolescent: 60–100 bpm	60–100 bpm
Respiration (R)	Respirations per minute (rpm)	Newborn: 30–50 rpm Infant: 20–30 rpm 2–12yrs: 20–30 rpm Adolescent: 12–20 rpm	12–18 rpm
Oxygen saturations (SpO$_2$)	Percentage %	99–100%	95–100%

Table 3.1: Vital signs and normal parameters

Activity 3.12

(a) Using the observation chart (Figure 3.3), write down the readings for all of Mr Devises' vital signs taken on 1 November 2010 at 02.00.

(b) For each vital sign determine whether it falls within acceptable parameters.

You may wish to compile your answer in a table with column headings: 'Date', 'Time', 'Vital sign reading' and 'Normal/abnormal'.

An outline answer is provided at the end of the chapter.

Early Warning Scores (EWS)

The monitoring of vital signs is part of a system that can alert you to an actual or potential deterioration in your patient's condition. The EWS is a tool used to evaluate a patient's health condition based on five physiological parameters: temperature, pulse, respiration, blood pressure and a responsiveness score. Points are allocated to readings that fall outside the normal parameters, thus alerting staff to a deterioration in the patient's condition. An overall score of three or above generally indicates that the patient requires an immediate medical review. The proper use and interpretation of an EWS and subsequent care intervention can help to reduce morbidity and mortality in acutely ill patients. It can also prevent patients deteriorating to the point where they need to be transferred to Intensive Care Unit (ICU) settings. Several types of EWS systems exist, so you should familiarise yourself with the one in use in your Hospital Trust when you start your next learning opportunity. It is important to remember that you must first be able to accurately measure, record and interpret your patient's vital signs before you can use an EWS.

This section has explored the use of observation charts and how they should be completed, and detailed the normal parameters for patients' vital signs. The next section will focus on the importance of calculating the correct doses of medicines.

Understanding medicine doses

While the whole process of medicines management is the responsibility of a variety of members of the multidisciplinary team, it is generally the nurse who has the responsibility for actually giving the medicines to the patient. The administration of medicines is a task nurses perform many times each day. It is therefore essential that nurses are able to calculate medicine dosages accurately. Only registered nurses can independently administer medicines – it is a skill that takes a lot of time, practice and experience to develop. So as a nursing student you need to use every opportunity to practise the skills involved in the administration of medicines under the direct supervision of a registered nurse.

When performing calculations, it is important that you understand what you are doing. Always ask yourself if the dose you calculate is a sensible one; estimate whether it is a likely answer. If you are unable to perform medicine calculations accurately, and consequently give the wrong dose of medication, this could have dire consequences for your patients. Never rely on the doctor or pharmacist to have got it right: everyone can make mistakes. Becoming familiar with some common formulas to calculate medicine dosages will help you in maintaining safe practice in medicine administration. This section will explore common units of measurement and weight used in medicines administration and the formulas required to calculate medicine doses and convert to different units of measurement and weight.

The International System of Units

The International System of Units, or Système International d'Unites (SI), is the metric system (also known as the decimal system) used to measure weights, volumes and lengths. It has been used in the NHS since 1975. The SI system is based on multiples of '10' and fractions of '10'. Prefixes are added after each basic unit to denote whether the units are larger or smaller than the basic unit. Table 3.2 shows the prefixes used to identify the size of a unit in multiples of 10. It is important that you are familiar with this system of measuring since you will use it on a regular basis when dealing with medicine doses.

Prefix	Numerical value
mega	1,000,000 (one million)
kilo	1,000 (one thousand
hecto	100 (one hundred)
deca	10 (ten)
deci	0.1 (one tenth)
centi	0.01 (one hundredth)
milli	0.001 (one thousandth)
micro	0.000001 (one millionth)
nano	0.000000001 (one billionth)

Table 3.2: Prefixes used in SI

Units and equivalences: units of weight and volume

Medicines – in tablet, liquid or powder form – have their strength expressed in units of weight or volume, using the SI system discussed above. Tablets and powder forms of medicines are generally expressed in terms of weight (for example, micrograms, milligrams or grams). Liquids are generally expressed in terms of volume (for example, millilitres or litres). They can also be expressed by moles or millimoles.

It is important to be familiar with how medicine strengths are expressed. It is also vital to know what their equivalences (alternative measurements) are. This is necessary because many times a day nurses need to administer to patients prescribed medicines where the dosage (strength) is prescribed in a different measurement from that supplied by the pharmacy department. It is necessary to know the common units of strength, their abbreviation and their equivalences. These are detailed in the table below.

Unit	Abbreviation	Equivalent	Abbreviation
1 kilogram	kg	1000 grams	g
1 gram	g	1000 milligrams	mg
1 milligram	mg	1000 micrograms	mcg*
1 microgram	mcg	1000 nanograms	ng*
1 litre	l or L	1000 millilitres	ml
1 mole	mol	1000 millimoles	Mmol
1 millimole	Mmol	1000 micromoles	Mcmol

Table 3.3: Metric units and their equivalents

*Please note that it is recommended that micrograms and nanograms should not be abbreviated, to avoid mistakes; that is, using the symbols 'mcg' and 'ng' (BNF, 2010).

There may be occasions when you see the abbreviations 'mcg' and 'ng' in books, journal articles or even on patients' prescriptions. You must always follow your Hospital Trust's policy regarding the approved abbreviations allowed to be used. It is rare for adult patients to have medicines prescribed in nanograms (ng) or micromoles (mcmol) but commoner for children because they have smaller dosages. Note that when dealing with plurals in a symbol the 's' is not included (write 2mg and not 2mgs).

Converting units

Each unit of strength (this can be either a weight, such as grams or micrograms, or a volume, such as litres or millimoles) differs from the next strongest or next weakest one by multiples of 1000. This means that to convert one strength to another you should multiply or divide by 1000. So, to express strength in a lower unit of measurement multiply by 1000 and to express strength in a higher one divide by 1000.

Worked example

You are asked to calculate how many micrograms there are in 1 milligram.

To do this, simply multiply 1 milligram by 1000, so:

1 x 1000 = 1000 micrograms

There are 1000 micrograms in 1 milligram.

You are asked to calculate how many litres there are in 1 millilitre.

To do this, divide 1 millilitre by 1000, so:

1 ÷ 1000 = 0.001 litre

There are 0.001 litres in 1 millilitre.

When carrying out medicine calculations it is always easier, and hence safer, to work in whole numbers. For example, when giving 0.5 litres of a medication, convert this into millilitres to get a whole number:

0.5 × 1000 = 500ml.

It is vitally important to move the decimal point the correct number of places (three places in this case) to prevent the administration of an incorrect dose to the patient.

Try the following exercise to test your understanding of units, weights, volumes and their equivalences.

Activity 3.13

Convert the following. Remember to include the correct units (where appropriate) in your answers.

(a) 5 milligrams into micrograms
(b) 20 grams into milligrams
(c) 10 litres to millilitres
(d) 3 moles into millimoles
(e) 0.6 litres into millilitres

The correct answers are provided at the end of the chapter.

Medicine concentrations or strengths

Medications are manufactured in many forms, including tablet, liquid, powder, spray and cream. There are several ways of expressing the concentration or strength of a medicine present in a medication preparation. When dealing with medicines in their liquid form, the most common way is to state milligrams (mg) of the medicine per millilitre (ml), expressed as mg/ml. The strength of other medicines might be expressed as micrograms per millilitre (ml) or nanograms per millilitre (ml). For example, the pharmacist stocks metoclopramide 5mg/ml and digoxin 100 micrograms/ml. Medicine prescriptions should state the strength of the medicine to be given rather than the volume of the liquid or the number of tablets. This is because different strengths can be manufactured for the same medicine. For example, flucloxacillin, for oral use, is manufactured in 250mg and 500mg capsules. It is also manufactured in syrup form at 125mg/5ml and 250mg/5ml. Examples of how prescriptions should be written can be seen in Figure 3.4.

Another way to express concentrations of medicines is by percentage concentration. Percentage concentration means the amount of the active drug in 100 parts of the product. The active drug can be in solid or liquid format and the product it is added to can also be in either solid or liquid format. So, when a solid has been dissolved in liquid, the percentage concentration refers to the number of grams (solid drug by weight) that have been dissolved in 100ml (volume of liquid). The abbreviated term used to express the percentage concentration is '% w/v'. The 'w' refers to the weight of the drug (for example, 10mg) and the 'v' refers to the volume of liquid it has been dissolved in (this will always be 100ml).

Percentage concentrations may also be expressed as the number of grams of a drug in 100g. This means that a drug has been added to another solid product. So to express the percentage concentration of a drug that has been added to another solid product, the expression '% w/w' is used, meaning (weight per weight, in this case) number of grams in 100g.

SURNAME Abdi	FORENAME Rahman	DATE OF BIRTH 12/07/2003 7 years and 5 months	PATIENT IDENTIFICATION NUMBER 290900	ALLERGIES None known
HEIGHT 1.2m	WEIGHT 21kg	CONSULTANT Saiko	SPECIAL DIETARY REQUIREMENTS None	

ONCE ONLY DRUGS/VARIABLE DOSE PRESCRIPTIONS

Date	Drug	Dose	Route	Prescriber's signature	Administered by	Date and time	Pharmacy

REGULAR PRESCRIPTIONS

		Time	Date

Drug Amoxicillin				06.00

Route O	Dose 125mg	Start Date 12/10/10	End Date 17/10/10	14.00

Prescriber's Signature R Halls		Pharmacy		20.00
				24.00

Drug Paracetamol				06.00
				12.00

Route O	Dose 250mg	Start Date 12/10/10	End Date 17/10/10	18.00

Prescriber's Signature R Halls		Pharmacy		24.00

Drug Bisacodyl				08.00

Route O	Dose 5mg	Start Date 12/10/10	End Date 17/10/10	

Prescriber's Signature R Halls		Pharmacy		20.00

Figure 3.4: A prescription chart

Finally, another way to express percentage concentrations is where a specific volume (for example, millilitres) of a medicine has been added to another liquid product. The percentage concentration is expressed as the liquid amount of the medicine added to another liquid product. This can be written as '% v/v' meaning volume per volume or number of ml in 100ml.

Calculation of medicine dosages

To ensure the correct amount of a medicine is given to each patient, you have to apply the basic principles of maths in order to calculate the correct dosage. You also need to be competent and feel confident in your ability to convert units of weight and volume into their equivalences. (This is one of the most common sources of drug dose errors.)

Medicines to be administered in solid form

For medicines to be administered in their solid form, such as tablets or capsules, the basic formula to use for calculating the amount of a medicine to be given is:

$$\frac{\text{What you want}}{\text{What you've got}} \quad \text{or} \quad \frac{\text{Prescribed dose}}{\text{Stock dosage (what's in the bottle)}}$$

This means that the prescribed dosage needs to be divided by the stock dosage that is available.

When the prescribed dosage and the stock dosage are of different strengths it is necessary to convert one of them into the same strength, but still maintaining their unit equivalence. This means that the dosage calculation should be worked out in the same unit. This is where dosage conversion is necessary. It is best practice to try to avoid working with decimal points as serious errors can occur. Imagine the consequences of putting a decimal point in the wrong place. The patient could end up with ten, a hundred or even a thousand times too much of the medication. (We hear about the resulting tragedies too often in the news.)

Medicines to be administered in liquid form

When calculating the amount of a medicine to give in liquid form the following formula can be used:

$$\frac{\text{What you want}}{\text{What you've got}} \times \text{the volume it is in}$$

or

$$\frac{\text{Prescribed dose}}{\text{Stock dosage (what's in the bottle)}} \times \text{the volume of the stock dosage}$$

An easy way to remember this formula is using the mnemonic 'NHS':

N = Need
H = Have
S = Solution

So

$$\frac{\text{Need (N)}}{\text{Have (H)}} \times \text{Solution (S)}$$

Another sensible rule to follow when calculating medicine dosages is to consider if your answer looks unlikely; for example, if it requires you to administer a large number of tablets or volume of liquid. It is always useful to double-check a calculation if this happens in case it is inaccurate. Similarly, if a calculation suggests a very small amount of liquid dosage or splitting a tablet, it is worthwhile rechecking the calculation.

Try the following exercise to test your understanding of medicine dose calculations.

Activity 3.14

Calculate how much would you administer to your patient if they were prescribed:

(a) oramorph 5mg, stock dosage is 10mg/5ml
(b) amoxicillin 375mg, stock dosage is 125mg/1.25ml
(c) paracetamol 1g, stock dosage is 500mg tablets
(d) digoxin 0.125mg, stock dosage is 62.5microgram tablets
(e) thyroxine 75microgram, stock dosage is 25microgram tablets

The correct answers are provided at the end of the chapter.

Medicine dosages based on body weight and body surface area

There will be many times when medicine dosages have to be administered according to the weight of the patient, particularly in children, or the body surface area (BSA). Some medicine dosages are also calculated to take into account other parameters, such as renal function or age.

Medicine dosages based on body weight

Medicine dosages prescribed relative to body weight are always calculated according to the patient's weight in kilograms (kg). For example, the medicine will be prescribed as milligrams (mg) per kg, micrograms per kg, nanograms per kg and so on. In order to determine the correct dosage, multiply the prescribed dosage by the patient's body weight in kilograms.

Worked example

A patient is prescribed dexamethasone 150micrograms/kg. He weighs 8kg. The dose to be given is:

150 micrograms x 8 = 1200micrograms or 1.2mg

Medicine dosages based on body surface area (BSA)

The dosage of some medicines may be calculated on BSA, in square metres (m^2). BSA is calculated for certain medicines, such as cytotoxic medicines (those used to treat cancer). To determine the patient's BSA, their height and weight must be known. The BSA can be calculated using the following formula devised by Mosteller (1987):

$$m^2 \text{ (BSA)} = \sqrt{\frac{\text{height (cm)} \times \text{weight (kg)}}{3600}}$$

Case study

Your patient, Rhianna Preston, is to be prescribed a medicine based on her BSA. She is 90cm in height and weighs 13.2kg. You have to calculate Rhianna's body surface area.

Using the formula above, these parameters are placed as follows:

$$BSA = \sqrt{\frac{90 \times 13.2}{3600}} = \frac{1188}{3600} = 0.33$$

The next step is to find the square root ($\sqrt{\ }$) of 0.33. This is 0.574 m^2. It is easier and much quicker to work this out with a calculator using the following steps:

- *Input '0.33'.*
- *Then press the square root key (marked with the sign '$\sqrt{\ }$') .*
- *Finally, press the equal or total key (marked with the sign '=').*

You should get the result that Rhianna's BSA is 0.574 m^2.

Do ask a colleague to check your calculation.

There are many formulas that can be used to calculate the BSA; the Mosteller formula is a relatively quick and simple one to use. You may also come across the use of a **nomogram** to obtain a BSA. A nomogram is a graphical representation of numerical relationships. Parameters are plotted on each graph. A straight line is then drawn through each plotted parameter (height and weight). Where the line intersects with the BSA column, this indicates the body surface area. A nomogram will only provide an estimate of the BSA. The following shows an example of a medicine prescription based on BSA.

Worked example

Your patient Harley Myers is prescribed 75mg/m² of doxorubicin. He has a BSA of 1.7m²

continued overleaf . . .

continued . . .

> To calculate how much of the medicine Harley should have, multiply the required dosage by the BSA.
>
> 75 x 1.7 = 127.5
>
> Harley requires 127.5mg of doxorubicin.

Try the following calculations related to medicine dosages.

Activity 3.15

A prescription reads to administer:

(a) Furosemide 0.5mg/kg via the oral route. The patient weighs 15kg. How many milligrams should be given?

(b) Gentamicin 4mg/kg via the intramuscular route. The patient weighs 60kg. The stock dosage is 40mg/ml. How many milligrams should be given?

(c) Gentamicin 4mg/kg via the intramuscular route. The patient weighs 60kg. The stock dosage is 40mg/ml. The patient has been prescribed the dosage, divided into three doses per day. How many millilitres should be given each time it is due?

(d) Prednisolone 60mg/m² via the oral route. The patient has a BSA of 0.45m². How many milligrams should be given?

(e) Desmopressin 1000 nanograms via the subcutaneous route. The stock dosage is 4 micrograms/ml. How many micrograms and millilitres should be given?

The correct answers are provided at the end of the chapter.

This section has enabled you to apply the basic mathematical principles to calculating drug doses for a range of formats of medicines. It has also introduced you to some particular formulas that are used when prescribing medicines to children. If you have found any difficulty in the activities, you need to revise your basic arithmetic until you are confident in your understanding, accuracy and speed. The BBC Bitesize and the HEA Mathcentre online resources offer revision material that you can access to improve your skills. Website addresses can be found at the end of this chapter. The next section continues with the theme of calculations, but focuses specifically on intravenous fluids.

Intravenous fluids and medical devices

As a student nurse you will not be allowed to administer any intravenous medicines or fluids to your patients. However, you will be expected to recognise if an intravenous fluid or medicine is administered correctly and at the prescribed rate. This section will cover the formulas required to calculate the rate at which an intravenous fluid or medicine should be administered. It will also discuss the use of medical devices in calculating administration rates.

Calculating intravenous infusion rates

Administering intravenous (IV) fluid is one of the most common therapeutic techniques used in hospitals. It is used for a variety of reasons, such as correcting fluid and electrolyte imbalances or as a medium for the administration of medicines. There are three stages to working out the rate at which IV fluids are given. A rate is an amount per unit of time.

* Stage 1: How many millilitres per hour need to be given?
* Stage 2: How many millilitres per minute need to be given?
* Stage 3: How many drops per minute need to be given?

Intravenous fluids are administered using a piece of equipment called a 'giving set', also called an 'administration set'. A giving set is simply a long piece of tubing that allows the fluid to drain from the bag containing the intravenous fluid into the patient via a cannula (a small plastic tube inserted into the patient's vein; the plural is cannulae). There are several different types of giving sets and the number of drops required to deliver 1ml of fluid will vary with each type of giving set.

* A standard giving set for administering a crystalloid (such as normal saline or 5% dextrose) will be capable of holding 20 drops of fluid per millilitre.
* A standard giving set for administering a colloid (such as blood, blood products or plasma expanding agents) will be capable of holding 15 drops of fluid per millilitre.
* A microdrop giving set (commonly known as a burette or a paediatric giving set) can hold 60 drops per ml of crystalloid solutions.

Consider a typical intravenous infusion (IVI) prescription in the example below.

Case study

Your patient Rubina Kapour is prescribed 1 litre of normal saline to be administered over 8 hours.

Using the stages described above:

Stage 1:   1 litre = 1000 millilitres

1000 ÷ 8 = 125

Therefore Rubina requires 125ml of normal saline per hour.

continued overleaf . . .

---

continued . . .

Stage 2:   *125ml ÷ 60 seconds = 2.08 ml per minute.*

This means Rubina needs to receive 2.08ml of normal saline per minute

To be able to progress to Stage 3, the number of drops of fluid per millilitre needs to be calculated. Since we are infusing a crystalloid we will be using a standard giving set that is capable of holding 20 drops of fluid per ml. So:

Stage 3:   *Multiply millilitres per minute by drops per millilitre to arrive at how many drops per minute the infusion should be set to run at.*

$$2.08 \times 20 = 41.6 = 42 \text{ drops per minute}$$

Rubina's infusion should run at 42 drops per minute.

Put simply, the formula to calculate IVI drip rates is:

$$\frac{\textit{Drops per ml of the giving set} \times \textit{amount in ml to be infused}}{\textit{Total infusion time in minutes}}$$

Activity 3.16

Assuming that standard giving sets are being used, calculate the following. Give your answers in ml/hr and also drops per minute and round your answers to the nearest whole number.

(a) 500ml of 5% dextrose (a crystalloid solution) over 6 hours
(b) 350ml of blood (a colloid solution) over 3 hours
(c) 300ml of normal saline over 6 hours (using a standard paediatric giving set that is capable of holding 60 drops per ml)
(d) 1 litre of gelofusine (a colloid solution) over 5 hours
(e) 600ml of blood (a colloid solution) over 4 hours

The correct answers are provided at the end of the chapter.

Medical devices

Whenever possible, IVIs should be administered via an infusion pump, which is a medical device. This provides exact control over the rate that the fluid is running. Like all such machines, its accuracy depends on the correct information being inputted.

The Medicines and Healthcare products Regulatory Agency (MHRA), an executive agency of the Department of Health, is responsible for checking all medicines and medical devices are safe to use. All medicine errors that occur using medical devices should be reported to the MHRA. Over-infusion of medicines and fluids, which is reported frequently, often leads to patient harm or even death. Between 1990 and 2000 there were 1,495 errors reported involving medical devices in the UK (Medical Devices Agency, 2003). The majority of errors were classed as 'user error'. Common errors include setting the wrong infusion rate, inputting the wrong size if a syringe is used and incorrect configuration of the pump.

Activity 3.17

Research a news story where a patient received either the wrong dose of a medicine or intravenous fluid administered using a medical device. What happened to the patient and what went wrong with the medicine or fluid administration?

As this is a personal research activity, there is no outline answer provided.

This section has enabled you to understand how to calculate intravenous infusion rates based on the equipment you have selected. The next section will focus on some common sample tests and how these can be interpreted.

Interpreting specimen results

It is very common practice to take samples or specimens of patients' blood, urine, sputum, wound exudate, stool, and so on for laboratory analysis. Various tests are conducted in the laboratory to determine whether the samples are within or outside normal parameters. The results are prepared by the laboratory staff and presented in the form of numerical data for many of these samples. Variations in these parameters will help to identify the health status of your patients and influence the treatment they need to receive. It is therefore very important that you and other members of the healthcare team are able to accurately interpret the data presented and respond accordingly.

Blood samples are probably the most common type of specimen taken from a patient. There are a variety of tests that can be performed. One such test is to determine the Full Blood Count (FBC) of your patient's blood. Results from this test will assist in identifying whether, for example, your patient has an infection, is anaemic or suffers from a blood disorder. This section will specifically focus on the values of the components of blood that are commonly tested when determining your patient's FBC. Table 3.4 below lists these blood components and the normal parameters you would expect to see in a healthy adult.

It is vital that you are able to identify when your patient's blood results fall outside these normal parameters. Try the following activity to test your understanding and interpretation of blood test results.

Blood components	Parameters
Haemoglobin	Men: 13–18g/dL
	Women: 11.5–16g/dL
Platelets	150–400 × 10⁹/L
Mean cell volume (MCV)	76–96Fl
White blood cells (WBC)	4–11 × 10⁹/L
Neutrophils	2–7.5 × 10⁹/L
Lymphocytes	1.3–3.5 × 10⁹/L
Eosinophils	0.04–0.44 × 10⁹/L
Monocyte	0.2–0.8 × 10⁹/L
Basophils	0.01 × 10⁹/L

Table 3.4: Normal parameters for blood components in FBC.
Adapted from Scott (2009) and Castledine and Close (2007).

Activity 3.18

For the following questions decide whether the blood test result is within or outside normal parameters for each patient. Write down what the normal range is. If the result is outside of the normal range, what do you think might be wrong with the patient? You may wish to present your answer in the form of a table with the following column headings: 'Normal', 'Abnormal', 'Parameter range', 'Possible diagnoses'.

(a) Molly Jones, 22 years old: haemoglobin (Hb) 7g d/L
(b) Danesha Williams, 15 years old: white blood cell (WBC) count 17 × 10⁹/L
(c) Dan Waddle, 39 years old, haemoglobin (Hb)16g d/L, platelets 300 × 10⁹/L

The correct answers are provided at the end of the chapter.

Other common blood tests include arterial blood gas analyses (ABGs); liver function tests (LFTs), urea and electrolytes (U&E), cardiac enzymes and lipids. This section has explored some of the common values for blood components and how interpretation of these values can aid a medical diagnosis and care interventions.

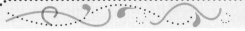

Chapter summary

This chapter has explored a variety of ways in which numerical skills can be applied to enhance nursing care. From reading this chapter you will have refreshed your understanding of basic calculation skills. You have been introduced to how numeracy skills can be applied to ascertain the health status of your patients, with particular focus on fluid balance and nutritional status. The chapter has discussed how to interpret patient data recorded on a variety of graphs and charts. You are aware that accurate interpretation and a thorough understanding of what this data means will determine the care and treatment your patients receive. Risk assessment has also been discussed, particularly in relation to nutritional status and the risk to a patient of developing pressure ulcers. Understanding and calculating medicine doses and intravenous infusion rates are crucial areas of patient care that can have dire consequences if not performed accurately; these has been covered in-depth in this chapter. Interpreting specimen results relating to blood samples have also been explored. Completion of the activities and undertaking additional reading into these important areas of nursing care where numeracy skills are required will assist you in acquiring the necessary proficiency for working and learning in your specific field of nursing.

Activities: Brief outline answers

Activity 3.1 (page 43)

(a) 75
(b) 33
(c) 25
(d) £22,850
(e) £9025

Activity 3.2 (page 43)

(a) 1152
(b) 2260
(c) 928
(d) 32
(e) 91

Activity 3.3 (page 44)

(a) 1 4/15
(b) 1 1/4
(c) 11/40
(d) 8/15
(e) 29/36

Activity 3.4 (page 45)

(a) 1/8
(b) 1/9
(c) 2 2/3
(d) 2 2/3
(e) 1/8

Activity 3.5 (page 45)

(a) 0.05
(b) 1.64
(c) 56.64
(d) 6.33
(e) 0

Activity 3.6 (page 46)

(a) 0.5
(b) 0.33
(c) 0.44
(d) 1/4
(e) 1/2

Activity 3.7 (page 46)

(a) 30
(b) 35
(c) 50%
(d) 99%
(e) 21%

Activity 3.8 (page 48)

(a) Hannah, 4 years
    James, 20 years
(b) 16 Health Care Assistants
(c) 150, 120, 90 students respectively

Activity 3.9 (page 51)

(a) Input = 1600ml; Output = 1275ml
(b) Positive balance of 325ml

VALLEY HILLS NHS FOUNDATION TRUST

PATIENT NAME:	HOSPITAL NUMBER:	DATE OF BIRTH:	WARD:	CONSULTANT:
Benji Todd	120967	12/12/2004	Oak	Roberts

DATE:

TIME	INPUT			OUTPUT		
	ORAL	I.V	I.V	URINE	VOMIT/NG	DRAIN
01.00						
02.00						
03.00		50				
04.00		50				
05.00		50				
06.00	75	50				
07.00		50		525		
08.00		50				
09.00	250	50				
10.00	100	50				
11.00		50				
12.00	150	50				
13.00	150					
14.00						
15.00	150					
16.00						
17.00						
18.00	150				100	
19.00						
20.00	125					
21.00						
22.00						
23.00						
24.00				650		
TOTALS (ml)	1100	500		1175	100	
TOTAL (ml) INPUT/OUTPUT	1600			1275		
FLUID BALANCE POSITIVE/NEGATIVE	325 ml positive					

Activity 3.11 (page 54)

Here are some numerical risk assessments you may have considered:
MUST tool: nutritional assessment
Waterlow tool: pressure ulcer risk

Activity 3.12 (page 57)

(a) and (b)

Date	Time	Vital sign reading	Normal/abnormal
1st November 2010	02.00	BP 125/75mmHg	Normal
1st November 2010	02.00	T 38.4°C	Abnormal
1st November 2010	02.00	P 65bpm	Normal
1st November 2010	02.00	R 22rpm	Abnormal

Activity 3.13 (page 61)

(a) 5000 micrograms
(b) 20000mg
(c) 10000ml
(d) 3000mmol
(e) 600ml

Activity 3.14 (page 64)

(a) 2.5ml
(b) 3.75ml
(c) 2 × 500mg tablets
(d) 2 × 62.5microgram tablets
(e) 3 × 25microgram tablets

Activity 3.15 (page 66)

(a) 7.5mg
(b) 240mg
(c) 2ml
(d) 27mg
(e) 1 microgram, 0.25ml

Activity 3.16 (page 68)

(a) 83ml/hr, 28 drops per minute
(b) 117ml/hr, 29 drops per minute
(c) 50ml/hr, 50 drops per minute
(d) 200ml/hr, 50 drops per minute
(e) 150ml/hr, 37 drops per minute

Activity 3.18 (page 70)

Normal/abnormal	Normal parameter range	Possible diagnosis
(a) abnormal	11–13g/dL	Anaemia
(b) abnormal	4–11 × 10⁹/L	Infection
(c) normal	Hb: 13–18g/dL	
	Platelets:150–400 × 10⁹/L	N/A

Further reading

Coben, D and Atere-Roberts, E (2005) *Calculations for Nursing and Healthcare*, 2nd edition. Hampshire: Palgrave Macmillan.

This concise book explains how to apply mathematical principles and numeracy skills to a variety of nursing care interventions.

Lapham, L and Agar, H (2009) *Drug Calculations for Nurses: A step by step approach*, 3rd edition. London: Hodder Arnold.

An easy-to-read book that explains the practical application of the mathematical principle needed for accurate medicine calculations.

Starkings, S and Krause, L (2010) *Passing Calculations Tests for Nursing Students*. Exeter: Learning Matters.

This book helps new nursing students succeed first time in medicines calculations tests, and get calculations right in practice. It takes the fear out of maths, even for those who find it a struggle, through clear step-by-step explanations and lively examples.

Useful websites

http://labspace.open.ac.uk

The Open University (OU) OpenLearn website gives free access to learning materials from higher education courses. To access this site registration is required, but it is free of charge.

www.bbc.co.uk/schools/ks2bitesize/maths/number

The BBC Bitesize online resources offer revision material that you can use to enhance your understanding of basic mathematical principles.

www.bnf.org/bnf

This site provides access to the online British National Formulary where information on clinical conditions, medicines and their preparations can be reviewed. Please note, user registration is required, although this is free of charge.

www.bnfc.org/bnfc

This site gives access to the online British National Formulary for children where information on clinical conditions, medicines and their preparations can be reviewed. Please note, user registration is required, although this is free of charge.

www.mathcentre.ac.uk/students.php/health/arithmetic

www.mathcentre.ac.uk/students.php/health/arithmetic/rules/resources

Another free useful online resource is the Higher Education Academy Centre for Excellence in Teaching and Learning Mathcentre, which offers students quick reference guides, practice and revision materials, video tutorials, workbooks and online practice exercises on many branches of mathematics.

Chapter 4
Working with others: interpersonal and communication skills

Nicola Davis

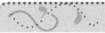
NMC Standards for Pre-registration Nursing Education

This chapter will address the following competencies:

Domain 2: Communication and interpersonal skills

Generic standard for competence

All nurses must use excellent communication and interpersonal skills. Their communications must always be safe, effective, compassionate and respectful. They must communicate effectively using a wide range of strategies and interventions including the effective use of communication technologies. Where people have a disability, nurses must be able to work with service users and others to obtain the information needed to make reasonable adjustments that promote optimum health and enable equal access to services.

All eight competencies for this domain are relevant to this chapter.

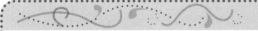
NMC Essential Skills Clusters

This chapter will address the following ESCs:

Cluster: Care, compassion and communication
6. People can trust the newly registered graduate nurse to engage therapeutically and actively listen to their needs and concerns, responding using skills that are helpful, providing information that is clear, accurate, meaningful and free from jargon.

By the first progression point:
1. Communicates effectively both orally and in writing, so that the meaning is always clear.

By the second progression point:
6. Uses strategies to enhance communication and remove barriers to effective communication minimising risk to people from lack of or poor communication.

continued overleaf . . .

continued . . . .

Cluster: Organisational aspects of care

9. People can trust the newly registered graduate nurse to treat them as partners and work with them to make a holistic and systematic assessment of their needs; to develop a personalised plan that is based on mutual understanding and respect for their individual situation, promoting health and well-being, minimising risk of harm and promoting their safety at all times.

Chapter aims

By the end of this chapter, you should be able to:

- understand why it is so important for nurses to continually develop their interpersonal skills;
- understand the range of verbal and non-verbal cues that help us communicate effectively with each other;
- explore how developing interpersonal skills can help both the therapeutic relationship and working relationships.

Introduction

Case study

Luca is just about to leave school and is considering his career options. He has found it stressful being at school because he feels quite shy and does not find it easy to socialise with strangers. Yet he imagines that he would like to do a job where he can help people. He goes to see the school careers adviser and discusses how he might overcome his shyness in order to be able to work effectively with other people. The careers advisor suggests that Luca joins a special interest group or even applies for a part-time job in a small shop. In this way, he might develop his ability to interact with other people.

One of the most important key skills that all nurses need to develop is the ability to communicate effectively with all of the people with whom you work. This requires well-developed interpersonal skills (IPS). When you applied for your nursing course, you communicated with academic staff who wanted to know why you applied. You are now forging new working relationships during your studies with peers, staff and, most importantly, clients. This starts within theory modules, but will enter a new level when you go into practice, when you will be dealing with new working pressures.

Nurses have a key co-ordinating role within healthcare and are frequently directly involved in the delivery of care. So how you interact with patients (service users or clients) is crucial to how the therapeutic relationship develops. Patients may very well judge nurses by how well they communicate. They quite rightly expect you to be approachable, friendly and able to communicate effectively with them. It can be a major source of complaint when you fail to communicate effectively. This is an expectation reinforced by the NMC, which recognises how important nurses' behaviour is in all the work that they do.

In this chapter we consider some of the main ways of effective communication. These include considering how to manage your own modes of communication and how to interpret these in other people. We will also look at assertiveness skills, how to deal with people you find difficult, and how to see things from the perspectives of the people that you care for. It is vital that nurses manage their interpersonal skills so as to be, and appear, reassuring to patients, to be patient advocates, and to progress the nursing process well. These skills will also help in working co-operatively within the interprofessional team.

Why nurses need to develop their interpersonal skills

Nurses are in a key position to build the therapeutic relationship. Everything that they contribute to care packages is built upon a foundation of effective communication. You need to be able to effectively assess, plan, deliver and evaluate care packages, all essential components of the nursing process, working with patients in partnership (DH, 2006). The nursing role is often quite pivotal in co-ordinating diverse care packages, some of which are individually tailored to patient needs. This requires the ability to listen effectively to clients, offer appropriate advice and develop the ability to be reassuring.

Sully and Dallas (2005) cite Rogers (1957) regarding the core qualities needed to build an effective therapeutic relationship. Warmth and genuineness are important because you need to be open and approachable to those for whom you care. You should appear credible and trustworthy in order to inspire the confidence of the patient. Unconditional non-judgemental positive regard is a very important concept to remember because nurses should not stereotype or be prejudiced against any particular client groups. Nurses should be accepting of difference and sensitive to cultural diversity. You should offer insightful assessment, plan and deliver effective care. This involves working with the client but should not involve judging them. Empathetic understanding is also vital and involves considering the 'patient's world' from their perspective. This last point is extremely important and worthy of closer exploration.

Scenario

Imagine you are a cyclist who has been riding to work, has gone over a large pothole and fallen off your bicycle. You are lying by the side of the road, shocked, upset and injured. Two strangers come down different sides of the road and both offer to help. They deal with the situation in very different ways.

continued overleaf . . .

continued . . .

One is a sympathetic person who sits down next to you, expresses how sorry they feel for your misfortune and may even quietly weep with you. The other stranger is an empathetic person. They appear to be far more 'in tune' with your predicament. They clearly assess the situation and sense you need more than sympathy, as you are in pain and in need of direct care and attention. They call for an ambulance, and stay with you to offer comfort as you wait because they understand that you should not be alone. They may realise you feel exposed and embarrassed so they put a coat around your shoulders and ask bystanders to move on.

It is empathy, rather than sympathy, that you need to develop and display as a nurse. This level of insight helps the care offered to be more tangible and effective. You offer the best care when you make every effort to understand the client's perspective, including what matters to them and what their priorities might be. Nurses can learn a lot from counselling theory and the following quote from Carl Rogers really reinforces the above point.

When functioning best, the therapist is so much inside the private world of the other that he or she can clarify not only the meanings of which the client is aware but even those just below the level of awareness. This kind of sensitive, active listening is exceedingly rare in our lives.
(Rogers, 1980, p116)

It should not be rare in nursing. This high level of professional insight may only be developed through an ongoing mutually beneficial therapeutic relationship that has been developed over a period of time. Nurses are not counsellors, unless they also complete a recognised programme of study, but you can usefully employ some fundamental counselling skills within your work. Understanding such skills helps you to see how you impact on social situations and what you can do to manage that in order to offer effective care.

Burnard (1995), a well-known key author who writes about communications skills, cites the work of Gerard Egan. Egan's theories have been highly influential within counselling theory. He designed a simple but effective prompt to help you to think about how you place yourself within a therapeutic situation. The mnemonic SOLER refers to five principal 'micro skills' that enable the management of your non-verbal cues within the therapeutic relationship. SOLER is defined in the box below.

Theory summary: SOLER: the five principal micro skills

- **S**itting squarely in relation to the client
- **O**pen posture
- **L**eaning slightly forward
- **E**ye contact
- **R**elax

Let's look at each of these principles in turn. First, you should consider how you position yourself when, for example, you complete a client's health needs assessment. You should sit squarely to the patient and close, yet not encroaching on their personal space. To get too close might make the client feel uncomfortable. It is also important not to appear confrontational, so it may be better to sit slightly to the side of them rather than directly in front. Bearing in mind that you can look very guarded if you cross your hands, or distant if you sit behind a table, it is important to appear appropriately open and therefore approachable. Leaning slightly forward can convey authentic interest in the other person, while being careful not to be too close. Eye contact is important to show genuine interest and authenticity. Be careful that eye contact is not staring, which can come over as confrontational, stressed or even aggressive. Appearing relaxed and not rushed should again show that you are paying due care and attention to the other person, maintaining focus on them, with enough time allocated to the planned interaction.

Using the SOLER skills you may already be well on the way to managing yourself within the therapeutic relationship. We will look at that self-management in more detail now.

Activity 4.1   *Communication*

Get into a pair with a friend or peer at university and find a quiet part of the room. Try recounting an important event to your partner while they apply the SOLER principles while they are listening to you. Then try the same activity but reverse the roles. How do you feel? Discuss your experiences and feelings when you have completed the activity.

An outline answer is provided at the end of the chapter.

The constituents of interpersonal skills

You might be surprised to know that the words you use in an interaction account for quite a small percentage of the total impact of your message. The words you use are delivered within a complex context that includes your body language (non-verbal cues) and tone of voice. Your non-verbal cues can make up approximately 70 per cent of the messages that you communicate. Tone of voice can account for approximately 23 per cent and the words you use can often account for only around 7 per cent of the message that you convey.

Scenario

You are talking to a friend, Anjoti, on the telephone. You ask her how her mother is and if she is feeling any better as you know she has not been well. There is a short silence on the other end of the telephone. Anjoti then tells you that she's doing okay thanks, and then changes the subject quickly to a night out planned that weekend. Reflecting on the conversation afterwards, you think that Anjoti sounded rather falsely bright about the weekend plans and you feel that she just wasn't quite her normal self. When you meet Anjoti at the weekend she confesses that her mother has had to go for a bowel cancer test and Anjoti didn't want to say anything on the telephone as she was still in shock about it.

When you talk to someone over the telephone, you can only hear them rather than see them as well. Yet we can give ourselves away with the tone of our voice and sometimes also in the pace of our speech. If someone stalls or stumbles over what they have to say or indeed sounds stressed, you might wonder why. If asked a difficult question that you don't want to answer, you might pause. However if an answer was forthcoming but conveyed in an unusual tone, as in the above scenario, that might raise concerns about the authenticity of the reply.

Communication needs to be a two-way process and through learning how to communicate effectively, you also learn how to interpret cues. As a nurse you need to engage proactively in partnership, working with clients and the interprofessional team to effectively interpret patients' verbal and non-verbal cues. You also need to learn how to manage you own cues, which we will now look at in turn.

Verbal cues

Verbal communication involves the use of the spoken word. Within nursing, there are times when verbal communication is particularly important – for example, nursing handovers, ward rounds, and health needs assessments when clients are admitted to clinical areas or teams. Verbal communication often has a written equivalent, such as documentation in the form of nursing admission notes and care plans. Nurses can make use of various verbal communication strategies to develop therapeutic relationships. A good example of this is paraphrasing some of the most important facts that clients have told you, showing that you are genuinely listening to them and checking with them that you have understood correctly. Nurses use these strategies in order to gain accurate and authentic information, and to help provide effective information-giving to patients or peers. Through careful communication, nurses demonstrate professional compassion for other people.

Hogan et al. (2008) discuss some of the distinct constituents of verbal communication that arise from an understanding of communication theory. As well as specific content, this includes the pace, intonation and clarity of the message.

The *pacing* of verbal communication can be very important. The rhythm and speed by which verbal messages are conveyed has an impact on how, and indeed how much of, the message may be received. A rushed message might be hard to take in. A long drawn-out explanation might be confusing.

The *intonation* of verbal communication includes the pattern of pauses, tones and stresses, which can also influence how a message is received. It can indicate the emotional state of the sender and impact on the emotional response of the receiver. To pause too much may make you appear ill-prepared and indecisive. To raise your voice may be interpreted as an act of aggression. To speak too quietly may indicate that you are under-confident or nervous.

The *clarity* of the message is also highly important because clear, succinct messages are more likely to be understood than vague lengthy messages, which can lose their focus and cause confusion. Effective communication makes thoughtful use of words, making the messages clear. Within healthcare this includes avoiding the unnecessary use of acronyms, abbreviations or jargon, which nurses may come to know but should not expect clients to understand.

Attending to the *timing* and *relevance* of how we verbally communicate reminds us that messages need to be delivered in a timely manner – this means at a time when the receiver is interested in receiving the message. Nurses often have to pick their time wisely when conveying bad news. Let's consider a scenario to demonstrate that.

Scenario

Imogen has been admitted to an acute surgical ward to be prepared for a planned sterilisation. She is a very pleasant, quiet lady, who is understandably nervous about the impending surgery. The nurse in charge of the ward has prepared Imogen for the surgery and they have discussed whether she is still happy to go ahead with the procedure. A little later during the morning, one of the anaesthetists rushes in and shouts at the nurse in front of Imogen, saying that the workload in theatre is much too high and he will cancel 'the next case', which is Imogen. The nurse is shocked by the anaesthetist's lack of tact and inappropriate behaviour. Before proceeding to make a complaint to her line manager about the anaesthetist's bad communication, the nurse goes over to Imogen. She apologises for what Imogen has just heard and gently reassures her that she will find out when her surgery will be.

This scenario highlights the fact that nurses are often working within view and earshot of clients. This means that your behaviour, demeanour, even the consistency with which you communicate, is on display. It is hard to build a therapeutic relationship, but all too easy to lose someone's trust through one thoughtless act.

Non-verbal cues

Non-verbal communication is the process of communicating without words. It can also be called body language and is a very powerful part of interpersonal communication.

The *tone* or *pitch* used can constitute what can be called paralanguage. What impression do you immediately make if you are loud, shrill, muttering, monotonous, or inaudible? To be loud can convey excitement, but also be interpreted as aggressive. To mutter may give an impression of nervousness. To sound monotonous may convey boredom.

Body posture includes gestures and other forms of body movement. What do you make of a patient who will not move from a slumped position? They might be in pain or be depressed in mood. What do you think of a colleague who always turns her back when you appear? This may be interpreted as an act of passive aggression, which can easily be interpreted as rude.

Our very appearance is in itself a means of communication, including how we *dress* and access-orise our appearance. If a student nurse is scruffy and has hair over her eyes, will a patient trust her to do her job properly? She may not be able to make proper eye contact, and patients may feel she is unhygienic and disinterested.

How we *smell* can also be a form of communication – for example, body odour can be interpreted as a sign of laziness or poverty, but might actually relate to a glandular problem. Lingering tobacco smoke or even strong perfume could also be offensive to patients, who cannot escape it.

Bear in mind that for clients who feel nauseous strong smells, even if pleasant normally, might make them feel worse.

Our expectations of acceptable levels of eye contact might be culturally driven, but in most cultures we are socialised to expect a certain level of eye contact. Too little can look evasive, too much can appear aggressive or even rude. Notice what you are comfortable with. This may in fact depend on who you are with.

Most of us have an 'invisible space' around us, like a comfort zone of personal space. We are used to having some control over who touches us, when and under what circumstances. It is rare to be in a situation where you might readily touch a stranger. You might like to consider how nursing practice creates situations where nurses have to transcend some of those usual social expectations when they are involved in direct care. This needs careful management as very personal care may be required by the client and again will be easier if a relationship of trust has already been established. This should create a situation in which both parties feel more comfortable.

Scenario

Bella is a nursing student who is asked by her mentor to offer a bed bath to an elderly gentleman on the ward. This will be the first time that Bella has washed someone else. She is understandably nervous and slightly embarrassed as she has never seen an elderly man naked before. The mentor senses Bella's anxiety and guides her through the process. She tells Bella that she needs to talk to the client first, ask his permission and prepare fully to make sure that she has all the resources needed not only to complete an effective bed bath, but also to take extra towels to cover his body and keep him warm during the wash. Bella finds that by preparing well, and concentrating on how her patient is feeling, she forgets her own anxiety.

Reading verbal and non-verbal cues requires both confidence and practice. Being able to do this helped Bella's mentor to assess the situation and help her through a difficult time in her learning journey. There are rarely hard and fast rules about how to articulate information, and each individual communicates in subtly different ways. A patient may cross their arms and appear uncomfortable because they feel emotionally vulnerable, or because they feel defensive because you are going to find out that they are hiding something. Some patients may declare that they are not in pain, yet appear physically uncomfortable in the manner they are moving around or 'guarding' a part of their body. It takes practice and experience to develop confidence in being able to 'read' the signs that reveal how someone is feeling. In a two-way process of communication, we often read each other's cues simultaneously as the interaction unfolds.

Most nurse–client interactions can be compared with social interactions in that they can be dynamic, responsive, reactive and socially contextualised. *The primary mode of communication is talk enhanced with gestures, personal communication style and body language* (Bach and Grant, 2009). When involved in giving direct care it is important to remember that the patient may well be influenced by the way that the nurse behaves, which can reveal how they might be feeling about certain issues. By managing yourself, being mindful of what you are doing and how you communicate, you can unlock the potential for better ways of working, which may well pay dividends in the future.

Empathy with the patient

Some of the most important influences on our motivation to develop inter-personal skills are our own experiences as a service user. It can be very difficult to feel empowered when you are anxious, fearful or in pain. Many of us know how powerless and vulnerable you can feel when visiting a close relative who is acutely unwell. Try to always bear in mind how the patient or relative might be feeling when you are in practice. They may appear overly assertive and even aggressive but in most cases they probably actually feel very frightened and frustrated because they may sense that there is very little they can do to influence or help their loved one's experiences.

Nurses can and should be effective advocates not just for the client but also for their families when they are closely involved. In aspiring to be effective advocates for clients, nurses should develop their interpersonal skills so they consistently appear both approachable and reassuring. It is arguably just as important to involve and inform carers wherever possible and appropriate, even though the established duty of care is not with them. Family-centred care has become an example of proactive and responsive care that recognises the privileged, yet vulnerable position of informal carers.

John McCarthy described his experiences of the first few days of his incarceration when he was kidnapped in Lebanon in 1986. In a keynote speech at a Royal College of Nursing Congress, he talked about what it was like to be taken by his captors to a remote building, where he was confined in a small, dark and dirty room. It was quickly apparent that he would be expected to eat, drink, sleep and even eliminate within that small space. He was dependent on the guards on duty for any small resource, like water or even human contact. This experience was in many ways defined by a lack of control. In fact, John had to make use of some skilful strategies in order to survive incarceration for over five years. One of these involved trying to gain some control, however small, over his environment. While there are major differences between being kidnapped and being a patient, there are similarities: which is why John was invited to speak that day. This is a good time to reflect on what it might feel like being an in-patient on an acute ward.

Case study

Ian Mackenzie is a 48-year-old man who has been admitted to Nightingale Ward for a liver biopsy. He has a wife and two sons. He has recently developed diarrhoea and vomiting. As a precaution, stool samples have been taken and he has been moved to one of the isolation rooms within the ward. Once moved to this side room, Ian spends all of his time in this one small room, with the door shut. He is dependent on the staff to bring him drinks because he finds the tap water in the jug tepid and unpleasant. He has to use the commode in the room to eliminate and wait for staff to visit his room for it to be emptied, which sometimes does not happen very quickly. There is no television and visiting is restricted to two hours a day in the afternoon. The door is not locked but he has been told not to leave the room as he could put other patients 'at risk', which worries him a great deal and makes him feel guilty. With only a couple of old magazines to occupy his time, he feels increasingly lonely and bored. He wonders when this ordeal will come to an end.

Activity 4.2   *Reflection*

Compare the stories of John McCarthy and Ian Mackenzie. Note any similarities in these accounts despite the differences in setting, one clearly far more frightening than the other. Make notes on the key points of comparison.

An outline answer is provided at the end of the chapter.

Dr Lesley Perman-Kerr, a chartered psychologist who has counselled hostages, proposed (on the BBC *News*) that it is not surprising that as a result of experiencing the most stressful and difficult circumstances conceivable, *people feel infantilised, demeaned, they may be held in claustrophobic conditions – all of those things will eat away at the person and make them unsure.* Bearing in mind the psychological and social effects of isolation, you might like to spend some time thinking about how nurses might use their interpersonal skills to help patients like Ian Mackenzie cope with his 'clinically imposed' solitary confinement. Amid scarce resources and high workload, the risk is very real that Ian might feel, or actually be, forgotten at times. You might consider how you would feel if you were in a situation where you felt powerless to act and had little to do but wait. I wonder how slowly time would go by in those circumstances.

Activity 4.3   *Reflection*

Remember, or imagine, circumstances when a close family member was very ill. Were you worried for them? How high were your expectations of the level of care that they would receive? How did the experience make you feel?

An outline answer is provided at the end of the chapter.

Being respectful

It is helpful to think of the patient as a customer. Most patients have a clear idea of what to expect from nurses and indeed from healthcare generally. There is access to so much information through different media about patient rights and how to get what you need. Yet when people are ill, they are not necessarily in a position to assert those rights, which increases their frustration and anger. A patient is vulnerable, and the nurse has a role to play in safeguarding them – for example, when a nurse is promoting an effective care package for a patient and in doing so can help the patient to have their needs recognised by other members of the interprofessional team.

Clinical governance has really defined the landscape of consumer expectation, which has changed from requiring care delivery to being influenced by a political process that has told people to expect consistently high standards of care delivery. One risk of not meeting these expectations is that patients and carers, who are now more aware of their rights, make complaints. It is good practice right from the start to aspire to deliver the best care you can, within the resources you have. If those resources become too limited, it becomes the responsibility of the nurse-in-charge to identify, document and report it through their line management team. It is also important to have integrity and in ethical terms demonstrate veracity, which means being honest. Clients may well respond better to honest responses about when and how much you can help them.

Activity 4.4 — *Reflection*

Think about the last time you went shopping. How did you expect the store assistant to behave towards you when you went to the till to pay? How did you feel if they were abrupt or unhelpful? Did you feel motivated and able to complain about poor service?

An outline answer is provided at the end of the chapter.

Interpersonal skills in therapeutic and working relationships

Millard et al. (2006) state that: *In the nursing literature, the nurse–patient relationship is consistently said to be of fundamental importance in promoting patient participation in nursing care.* The success of this relationship depends on how well information is exchanged and how power is transferred from nurse to patient, and vice versa. It is the process by which a decision is reached that defines the approach to partnership. It is therefore important that interactions between nurse and client should be the central element in enabling patient participation in their nursing care. Nurses need to be approachable and trustworthy in order make this relationship work.

Activity 4.5 — *Reflection*

Think about the circumstances under which you would voluntarily self-disclose personal information. What would make that seem possible?

An outline answer is provided at the end of the chapter.

You may have found in your reflection that any self-disclosure would be far more likely to happen in a situation where you trusted, and felt comfortable with, the listener.

Establishing good practice: assessment on admission

As a nurse you will need to use your interpersonal skills to build the therapeutic relationship both efficiently and effectively. This is vital, particularly at the beginning of the nursing process when you assess the individual patient to establish their care needs. This is your opportunity to make a good first impression. In most circumstances the patient will be able to communicate in some way and usually, if given the time and opportunity, do so quite well. 'Tuning in' to the patient's perspective at that time allows you to identify exactly what is needed by them and for them. This is an important first opportunity to empower the patient, actively involve them and convey that they are genuine partners in directing their care.

The quality of the entire nursing process requires careful attention to detail at every stage. The initial assessment is the foundation upon which you can build clinically effective care packages. To encourage frank disclosure of information, you need to be, and appear to be, approachable, interested and authentic. To hear what the patient is saying to you, you need to be motivated and able enough to actively listen to them. It is therefore essential to have enough time to do so. You need to manage your non-verbal cues to show that you do have the time and motivation to focus on the patient, and listen to what they have to tell you. Remember to use the SOLER mnemonic (see page 78).

At this stage you are also building working relationships within the team. Make sure your documentation is of a high standard, as this will show not only that you have heard what has been said to you and recorded what you did, but also that you respect the need to communicate with the wider team of professionals who will be caring for the patient. You will also need to convey verbally what you have achieved during shifts in handovers.

To remind you of some of the core issues we have already discussed, here is a mindful mnemonic.

A mindful mnemonic

M = Measured: appear even-handed and non-hierarchical in your approach

I = Individualised: maintain focus on the individual client whenever appropriate

N = Non-judgemental positive regard: appear caring in a non-discriminatory, consistently fair and even-handed manner

D = Deal with challenges that you are sure you can handle and ask for help with any challenges that you know are beyond your current scope of practice

F = Fidelity: faithfulness to duty (of care) – remember the contractual expectation of accountability for what is and is not done

U = Understanding: consider the other person's perspective

L = Location: think about the environment in which you are communicating. Is it appropriate?

N = Needs: are the other person's needs being taken into consideration?

E = Emotional Intelligence: are you managing yourself and how you feel?

S = Safety: are you considering your own and the other people's safety in managing this situation?

S = Security: do you appear authentic and reassuring in the way that you are communicating with other people?

Assertiveness skills

There is a radical difference between being assertive and being aggressive. It is perfectly possible to remain professional while being assertive. You can be assertive while still respecting mutual rights, and perhaps to a lesser extent also wants and needs. Being assertive allows you to appreciate the other person's perspective, but also requires shared acknowledgement that you have rights too. In this chapter, we have considered how important it is for the patient to feel respected and listened to. It is also important to assert that you have rights too, including the right to be treated fairly and not be abused, verbally or otherwise. One problem you might occasionally encounter is that some physical and psychological conditions reduce the individual's capacity to express themselves appropriately – for example, when a patient has Alzheimer's disease, some types of infection or is recovering from some specific surgical procedures. You will learn how to deal with such challenges through observing how your mentors manage and defuse situations where a client's behaviour challenges the safety of staff or other clients.

A further potential problem might develop from being 'emotionally attached' or overly involved with some patients. Bach and Grant (2009) recognise this problem:

> *One of the concerns professionals often have is how to become involved with a patient in a sufficiently supporting manner without becoming over-involved and not being able to stand back and objectively assess the needs of the patient. Being oneself and bringing personal characteristics to the relationship is crucial, otherwise we would be very mechanical and would be like androids or robots giving care.*

With experience, healthcare professionals learn how to find that balance between making a connection, yet not transgressing safe boundaries. Two concepts that help with achieving that balance are emotional intelligence and dealing with difficult challenges, which we will look at now.

Emotional Intelligence

Goleman (2001) states that:

> *The rules for work are changing. We're being judged by a new yardstick: not just by how smart we are, or by our training and expertise, but also by how well we handle ourselves and each other.*

This is certainly true of nursing. Nurses are mandated through NMC professional regulation not only to act in the patient's best interests but also to work co-operatively. Emotional intelligence involves considering where and how you might manage your feelings in order to express yourself effectively.

Scenario

Imagine you are a young woman working in the community completing a leg dressing on a young man who has been in a car accident. He asks you to meet him socially 'after work'. You know that however much you might like him this is not the place from which to progress to dating. You need to find a way to politely decline, while trying to avoid causing distress.

Emotional intelligence involves knowing how to handle your emotions, what motivates you and how you can develop empathy. All of these issues are highly relevant when working in healthcare. Goleman (2001) states that in a national survey about what employers looked for in new employees, listening and oral communication were top of the list. How you manage your interpersonal skills will be directly linked with how you manage yourself more generally. First encounters can be very important, so you need to be organised and contact each practice experience setting before you start there. Remember, every interpersonal encounter can form an opportunity to impress.

Activity 4.6   *Decision-making*

You are on your first clinical experience opportunity in an acute ward. One of the patients is visibly upset about being kept waiting for several hours by the medical team who should by now have started doing their rounds. The patient is expecting to be discharged that day and wants to get on with the arrangements to go home. What can you do?

An outline answer is provided at the end of the chapter.

Dealing with challenge

This final section is about managing yourself within a pressured working environment. Developing resilience is one of the most important features for successfully completing pre-registration studies and forging a future within healthcare. Working within healthcare in the UK is demanding. The service is predominantly 'free at source' and often over-subscribed. There will almost always be more to do than resources can easily meet. When you are working within challenging and pressurised environments, it may be all too easy to default to routines and defensive practice where 'corners might be cut'. It can be very challenging to counter-balance delivering both quality and quantity of work. It requires strength of character and high expectations of you to manage working under pressure. Coping in the face of adversity and still communicating well is a benchmark of true professionalism, which all nurses have to develop.

Developing confidence is similarly very important. Confidence should be built upon a foundation of preparation, understanding and good practice. It is important to develop inner confidence in the face of challenge, which will occur at times. As you develop knowledge and understanding of both theory and practice underpinning effective interpersonal skills, you may develop confidence in your ability to communicate well.

Dealing with difficult people is a frequent challenge within healthcare. Thornton (2002) considers strategies for dealing with difficult colleagues. His ideas remind us of some of the fundamental messages within assertiveness training. Every individual has their own position, but as well as having rights, they also have responsibilities to respect the rights of others. Thornton describes three main types of work colleague: the aggressor, the victim and the rescuer. The first type can be particularly challenging because they have the potential to be forceful, demanding, intimidating and may bully other people. Victims can be defined by their reluctance to take responsibility, yet persist in blaming external agencies and individuals for their problems. The rescuer can be 'unconsciously incompetent', so busy 'helping' their colleagues that they do not complete their workload. Always be clear about what work has been allocated to you and how you can prioritise so that it is completed.

You also need to be prepared for clients, peers, colleagues or perhaps even managers who appear not to communicate well with you. Thornton (2002) cites some helpful strategies to consider using.

- Listen to the other person's point of view and actively try to hear what they have to say.
- Aim to appear as if you respect other people's right to their opinion and value them as people.
- Try to identify whether they have any awareness of what type of person they are and what roles they tend to 'play'. Try to identify if there might be a way to increase their self-awareness.
- Try to consider what their strengths and weaknesses are.
- Do you think it is possible for them to change?

On this last point, try to consider who or what might facilitate a change in the behaviour of challenging individuals. If you feel that a patient is being unpleasant to you, talk to your mentor or the nurse-in-charge about the issue and seek their advice. If it is a member of staff, be clear that you have the right to learn without fear of intimidation. When you go into practice, make sure that you have already identified and kept a note of the details of members of academic staff and practice staff who may be able to support you.

Conclusion

The Department of Health (2001) is very clear in asserting the central co-ordinating role of nurses within healthcare. From the very first health needs assessment through to the well-planned discharge, the nurse is pivotal in making sure that the patient is fully assessed, a care package is planned with them, quality care is delivered that matches expectations, and that care packages are evaluated with care and consideration. The whole of the nursing process is effectively enabled by well-developed interpersonal skills. The Department of Health (2006) defines communication as a process that incorporates meaningful exchange(s) between at least two people. These exchanges form a medium in which to convey facts, needs, opinions, thoughts and feelings. This two-way process involves the exchange of information through both verbal and non-verbal means, including face to face and the written word.

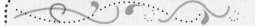

Chapter summary

This chapter has emphasised that developing your interpersonal skills will help you to develop your working relationships with patients, peers and practice staff. Through considering how cues can be well managed and conveyed, therapeutic rapport can facilitate and be facilitated by a trusting relationship between nurse and patient. This can help to make most working processes run smoothly. In times of challenge, these skills may also facilitate resolution in the midst of conflict and challenge as well.

Activities: Brief outline answers

Activity 4.1 (page 79)

SOLER is designed to convey a carefully pitched interest in the client, involving active listening. You should have felt that this interest was comfortable rather than intrusive. There may have been a difference in how each of you felt when you experienced being on the receiving end of this technique. You might want to reflect on how your expectations might be somewhat different if you were ill.

Activity 4.2 (page 84)

The key points of comparison are related to disempowerment, vulnerability, social and emotional isolation. A common experience of those people who have spent a period of time in isolation is a sense of loneliness. Human beings are predominantly social creatures. Perhaps you also discussed the potential vulnerability of clients, who might not feel as if they have very much control when they access healthcare. Clients need to feel empowered to participate in directing their care packages. The nurse therefore needs to feel able to be an effective advocate and be proactive in making sure that the client's needs are met.

Activity 4.3 (page 84)

Whenever one of my close relatives is in hospital I feel quite anxious. I hope that they are comfortable, receiving help when they ask for it and being treated with respect. If that were found to not be the case I would feel motivated to complain. Whenever I have been an in-patient myself I have felt that at least some of my care package was out of my hands and that felt quite frightening because most of us are used to being in control most of the time. Were your experiences similar or different? Don't worry if your experiences were different; we are all individuals. The important thing is to reflect on our experiences and see whether that insight can develop our understanding.

Activity 4.4 (page 85)

This is about your expectations of customer service. When I go into a shop I expect the assistant to be friendly, polite and able to answer my questions with courtesy and integrity. I expect to be sold something that is both safe, effective and fit for purpose. If there is a problem, I expect the assistant to politely and efficiently resolve the problem. I expect to be listened to, heard and treated with respect. I do not have to visit the shop and buy products there. The assistant is paid to be there because shoppers may want to visit the shop. It is very important not to alienate the customer. I would suggest that increasingly this will be the attitude of clients we care for.

Activity 4.5 (page 85)

Your answers might have included the qualities of someone who inspired your trust. You might need to be reassured regarding how confidentiality will be maintained regarding your personal information. You would probably want the individual gathering the information to be professional. You might have also added the issue of data protection as well, although this list is not exhaustive.

Activity 4.6 (page 88)

In this activity you are asked to consider how to deal with a patient who might be about to make a complaint, which understandably may make you feel nervous. As a very new student, your first and best option might be to politely excuse yourself, explaining that you are going to find the nurse in charge of the shift and ask them to come and discuss the issues with the patient. As you become more experienced, you might feel able to start a conversation with the patient, exploring what their grievances are. The simple act of listening to the patient's concerns and hearing what they have to say may help them feel a little better.

Ultimately, however, the situation will need to be more fully responded to – for example, by the nurse-in-charge contacting the medical team to find out when they are going to arrive on the ward and attend to this particular patient.

Further reading

Bach, S and Grant, A (2009) *Communication and Interpersonal Skills for Nurses.* Exeter: Learning Matters.

This is a good text focusing on IPS related specifically to nursing, written in an accessible style.

Department of Health (2006) *Chief Nursing Officer's Review of Mental Health Nursing: Summary of responses to the consultation.* London: HMSO.

This DH Review was established to explore ways in which mental health nurses could best participate in delivering care to and with people with mental health problems in the future NHS. As such, it is very revealing of some key professional issues related to interpersonal skills and the therapeutic relationship.

Goleman, D (2001) *Working with Emotional Intelligence.* London: Bloomsbury Publishing.

A very accessible text focused on applying emotional intelligence in the workplace.

Hogan, M, Bolten, S, Ricci, M and Taliaferro, D (2008) *Nursing Fundamentals.* New Jersey: Prentice Hall.

A good, broader text focused on nursing skills, often popular with current students due to its accessible style.

Sully, P and Dallas, J (2005) *Essential Communication Skills for Nursing.* London: Elsevier Mosby.

A good, broader text focused on communication skills.

Thornton, P (2002) *The Triangles of Management and Leadership.* Coral Springs, Florida: Llumina Press.

This text contains a more in-depth discussion about how to deal with difficult people. It is presented in a highly accessible and engaging style.

Useful websites

http://interpersonalskills.org/

www.learnhigher.ac.uk/Students/Listening-and-interpersonal-skills.html

Both of these websites contain a good range of additional information on interpersonal skills that you might enjoy studying.

Chapter 5
Being literate: writing skills for nursing practice

Alison C Clark

NMC Standards for Pre-registration Nursing Education

This chapter will address the following competencies:

Domain 2: Communication and interpersonal skills

3. All nurses must use the full range of communication methods, including verbal, non-verbal and written, to acquire, interpret and record their knowledge and understanding of people's needs. They must be aware of their own values and beliefs and the impact this may have on their communication with others. They must take account of the many different ways in which people communicate and how these may be influenced by ill health, disability and other factors, and be able to recognise and respond effectively when a person finds it hard to communicate.

7. All nurses must maintain accurate, clear and complete records, including the use of electronic formats, using appropriate and plain language.

8. All nurses must take every opportunity to encourage health-promoting behaviour through education, role modelling and effective communication.

Domain 3: Nursing practice and decision-making

8. All nurses must provide educational support, facilitation skills and therapeutic nursing interventions to optimise health and wellbeing. They must promote self-care and management whenever possible, helping people to make choices about their healthcare needs, involving families and carers where appropriate, to maximise their ability to care for themselves.

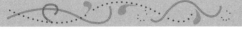

NMC Essential Skills Clusters

This chapter will address the following ESCs:

Cluster: Care, compassion and communication

6. People can trust the newly registered graduate nurse to engage therapeutically and actively listen to their needs and concerns, responding using skills that are helpful, providing information that is clear, accurate, meaningful and free from jargon.

Introduction

This chapter will help you explore how to write about your nursing practice clearly and succinctly. Knowing what and how to write information to suit the reader's needs is a core skill. Perhaps you have taken something you have written to a tutor, or another nurse, only to be told that you haven't explained yourself clearly. Sometimes we make assumptions that 'the reader knows what we mean'; that we don't have to state the obvious. Alternatively, have you been put off reading an article because of the unfamiliar language? Mentors and students, for instance, often complain that they cannot understand the requirements of the Nursing and Midwifery Council's outcomes and competencies (2004) because of the way they are worded (Clark, 2009). Last year I asked my personal students to give me feedback on my teaching. Some indicated that they found the way I explained things difficult to understand because I use unfamiliar terms such as 'rationale' and 'context'. They would prefer it if I could say things more simply. I realised that I have internalised, adapted to and adopted medical, nursing and educational terminology in my teaching.

What does 'being literate' mean?

There are many different definitions of, and types, of literacy (see concept summary box on p94). At its simplest it is the ability to *read and write* (Swannell, 1986). The NMC (2010a) requires all registered nurses to have *a good command of written and spoken English* (and, where appropriate, Welsh). This includes the ability to *Read and comprehend (in English or Welsh) and to communicate clearly and effectively in writing to include using a word processor* (NMC, 2008a, p3) and be able to *interpret and present information in a comprehensible manner* (NMC, 2007, p8). A public consultation defined a comprehensive list of literacy skills that need to be developed and assessed throughout pre-registration. These included understanding instructions and information, documentation skills, note-taking skills, form filling online, plus the addition of handwriting skills and effective use of these to transfer information (The Focus Group UK, 2007).

> ## Concept summary: three increasingly complex definitions of literacy
>
> **Literacy** = *Reading, writing, and the creative and analytical acts involved in producing and comprehending texts.* (adlit.org, undated)
>
> **Functional literacy** = *The ability to read, write and speak in English, and to use mathematics at a level necessary to function at work and in society in general.* (Easton et al., 2010)
>
> **Scientific literacy** *is the knowledge and understanding of scientific concepts and processes required for personal decision making, participation in civic and cultural affairs, and economic productivity. It also includes specific types of abilities; a person can ask, find, or determine answers to questions derived from curiosity about everyday experiences. It means that a person has the ability to describe, explain, and predict natural phenomena. Scientific literacy entails being able to read with understanding articles about science in the popular press and to engage in social conversation about the validity of the conclusions. Scientific literacy implies that a person can identify scientific issues underlying national and local decisions and express positions that are scientifically and technologically informed. A literate citizen should be able to evaluate the quality of scientific information on the basis of its source and the methods used to generate it. Scientific literacy also implies the capacity to pose and evaluate arguments based on evidence and to apply conclusions from such arguments appropriately.* (National Science Education Standards, undated, page 22)

Applied literacy skills, introduced as part of the Essential Skills Clusters from September 2008 for all pre-registration programmes (NMC, 2007a and b), are now embedded within the 2010 competencies (see Table 5.1). The expected levels of achievement are linked to two progression points, at the end of the foundation programme and at the end of branch.

Pheasey (2002), however, suggests that literacy is more than the ability to access information, read, write, comprehend information and spell correctly using a given language. People can 'be literate' in many different ways – socially, culturally, visually and geographically. Pheasey writes about 'streetwise' individuals who can find their way around town easily, and act as guides for others, without necessarily being able to 'read' a map or street signs; she calls this 'geographical literacy'. The notion of being literate therefore needs to be set within a given context (in the environment within which we live and work). In collating various definitions of literacy it would appear that literate people can:

- perceive the need for information;
- access information effectively by observing, listening, 'reading'* and appraising the value of information from a variety of sources (visual, auditory, sensory) that occur in a given social and cultural situation (context);
- understand the information (comprehend) and give it personal meaning in order to make sense of what is happening;
- apply information to new situations (where appropriate) and where necessary act accordingly;
- convey information to others using 'language' and media that are appropriate to the audience's needs (words, sounds, symbols, even modelling practices or behaviours suited to the situation).

* to define 'reading' in its broader sense also means to 'hear and listen to', 'see and watch', 'feel (Braille)', 'taste', 'smell' (e.g. sensory gardens or care environments), etc.

First progression point	Second progression point	Entry to the register
1 *Communicates effectively both orally and in writing, so that the meaning is always clear.* 2 *Records information accurately and clearly on the basis of observation and communication.* 3 *Always seeks to confirm understanding.* 4 *Responds in a way that confirms what a person is communicating.* 5 *Effectively communicates people's stated needs and wishes to other professionals.*	6 *Uses strategies to enhance communication and remove barriers to effective communication minimising risk to people from lack of or poor communication.*	7 *Consistently shows ability to communicate safely and effectively with people providing guidance for others.* 8 *Communicates effectively and sensitively in different settings, using a range of methods and skills.* 9 *Provides accurate and comprehensive written and verbal reports based on best available evidence.* 10 *Acts autonomously to reduce and challenge barriers to effective communication and understanding.* 11 *Is proactive and creative in enhancing communication and understanding.* 12 *Uses the skills of active listening, questioning, paraphrasing and reflection to support a therapeutic intervention.*

Table 5.1: Applied literacy skills progression points (NMC, 2010)

Plus, some definitions include being numerate.

'Being literate' in nursing

Many of the 2010 NMC competencies are underpinned by the need for sound literacy skills. These are illustrated in Table 5.2. On one hand, as a nurse you need to be able to communicate across different professional groups utilising discipline-specific 'professionally' orientated language common to all – for example, in co-ordination of recovery from illness and discharge planning. On the other hand, you need to understand and document how patients may express their health needs or signs and symptoms of illness in more colloquial language (Davies, 2010, Shears, 2010, Deigham, 2008). The latter becomes even more important when we consider that you often need to work through other people such as interpreters (preferably) or family members when communicating with patients. It is vital that you ensure that information is translated appropriately for informed consent to investigations, care and treatment when acting as a patient's advocate and when providing patient information and education. An understanding of literacy, and the factors that influence how individuals take on board and use written information, is also important in the development of 'written' patient information (Department of Health, 2003, 2008a). You need to be able to interpret and convey information in different ways for different audiences' needs, such as for those with a low level of literacy, the visually or hearing impaired, for those with cognitive impairment, as well as for our professional colleagues.

Case study

Gina recently worked with Miss Adams, a patient worried about future surgery and its potential effect on her health and well-being. First, Gina checked Miss Adams's understanding of her previous treatment and what she thought was going to happen next. In order to do this, Gina drew a diagram of the relevant anatomy and physiology and discussed with Miss Adams what she remembered about the effects of her previous treatment and the next stage. They looked at the terminology the nurses and doctors had used and clarified what it meant. Then they explored what she feared most, how to get more information and from whom (the relevant nurse specialists to contact, and how). Miss Adams seemed unaware of the different roles of the specialists involved, or that there were self-help groups that could help her manage her condition. Some of this may have been forgotten in her anxiety and influenced her ability to take information on board. However, nothing seemed to have been written down to help her remember the stages in her treatment plan, and who to contact. After spending about an hour talking to Gina, Miss Adams went away with a diagram to understand her condition, a list of people who could help and how to contact them, and felt reassured about contacting them.

The everyday language people use is determined by many factors – their upbringing, their culture, even sometimes where they live in the country.

Activity 5.1   *Communication*

Divide a piece of paper into two columns and complete this activity.

You are out and about with your friends when you realise you need to go to the toilet. Write down the words or phrase you use to tell your friends you are going to the toilet in the first column.

As a nurse, you often ask people if they have 'passed urine'. In the second column write down how you ask a patient if they need to use the toilet or have passed urine.

Now look at Table 5.2. Are there any similarities or differences to the ones you have come across?

Reflect on why we need to be aware that people might ask about going to the toilet using a variety of different words or phrases.

As this is a personal exercise, there is no outline answer provided.

Patient-orientated	Professionally-orientated
Communicate orally/in writing • Completing assessments, general and specific • Planning and writing care plans • Promoting self-care and self-management • Using different communication equipment • Patient information and education – diagrams, posters, leaflets, using the internet • Completing information prescriptions	**Nursing and multidisciplinary records** • Referral letters • Discharge letters • Case conference notes
Patient/carer participation • Recording effectiveness of given care • Evaluating care • Signposting to services • Referring care to colleagues	**Collaborate with others (team work)** • Handovers • Court reports
	Legislation • Consent • Mental competence

Table 5.2: The range of literacy skills that underpins the ESCs, including the ability to convey information through writing

As a first-year student nurse, I can remember an elderly male patient asking if he could go for a 'whiddle'. I didn't know what he meant, and he became very embarrassed when he had to explain it to me. It would have been useful if his word for 'passing urine' had been documented in his nursing notes. You might want to consider this when writing care plans. Do you use nursing or medical terminology or the patient's words to record your assessment of their needs, their usual behaviour and lifestyle preferences?

'Being literate' in nursing, at an individual patient care level, is fundamental to:

- listening to, appreciating and conveying ideas about what 'being healthy' means;
- helping people to
  - recognise what is healthy and what are signs and symptoms of illness
  - why attendance for immunisation or screening tests is important to protect their health, prevent illness or detect illness early
  - understand what investigations and procedures mean
- helping people to manage illness and/or become self-caring;

Professional	Lay	Colloquialisms
urinate micturate	go to the toilet pass water pass urine	wee/wee wee pee go to the loo number one spend a penny tiddle whiddle jimmy riddle go and see a man about a dog
dysuria	hurts when I pass water/urine stings when I pass water /urine	
haematuria	blood in my water/urine	
oliguria	not passing a lot of water	
anuria	not passing any water	
nocturia	go to the toilet during the night	getting up to the loo all night
polyuria	passing a lot of urine	weeing a lot

Table 5.3: Professional, lay and colloquial language: an example

- working with, and sometimes co-ordinating or leading, teams of healthcare professionals for holistic care.

Clinically, 'being literate' requires us to:

- recognise a need to enhance our understanding of a current patient situation in order to assess, plan, provide, review, audit, and perhaps change practice (i.e. determine how the context in which the care is occurring influences how we communicate; this is discipline-specific literacy);
- access information from a variety of sources in order to make sense of the patient's needs across clinical settings, i.e. as patients move between primary, secondary and tertiary care settings practice may differ;
- 'read' and interpret information in order to understand its value within a certain practice context in order to make appropriate clinical decisions (be a knowledgeable practitioner);
- interpret information with and for other people in order to convey ideas, information and decisions meaningfully, i.e. verbally or in writing, using a recognisable language (be a skilled practitioner);
- take responsibility for how, and what, information is recorded;
- make authoritative recommendations for practice.

Review point 4 in Table 5.1 and consider the following case study. How does Jane, a senior nurse, demonstrate a range of literacy skills?

Case study

Jane, a senior nurse, was setting up a cancer support group meeting. She noticed Ellen and Joanne arrive looking somewhat flustered. They had missed the bus and were late. She watched as group members gathered around and made sure they had a cup of tea and some sandwiches. Jane could tell that Ellen wasn't settling. Stan came over to Jane a few minutes later to say he was concerned about Ellen. She was worried she had forgotten to take her 'diabetic pills'. Jane told Stan she would sit with Ellen while the rest of the group started the meeting. Ellen was agitated. She told Jane she wasn't feeling well, and although she had 'had a bite' of the sandwiches she was feeling shaky and a bit sick. Holding Ellen's hand, Jane surreptitiously took Ellen's pulse, while listening to her. Her pulse was fast, thready and irregular. Jane asked Ellen if anything else was going on that she should know about. Ellen admitted to being worried she was 'having another heart attack' (it's been a year since her last one). She has been having chest pain on and off for the last few days and not settling, even after taking her GTN spray. Ellen was worried she would have to go back into hospital. Jane suggested they get some advice before she went home (Ellen is 83 and lives alone). Jane asked Ellen if it was okay for her to ring the local accident and emergency department. She asked Joanne to sit with Ellen while she made the call. Jane spoke to one of the A&E sisters. Both she and Jane felt Ellen must be seen in A&E rather than go home. Jane explained to Ellen that while she appreciated how frightened she was, it might be best to pop her round to A&E and get it checked out now (rather than her feel poorly when she got home).

Jane had picked up cues 'that there was something different' happening with Ellen: more than her just missing her pills. In nursing patients with similar conditions, over a period of time and perhaps in a variety of settings, Jane has internalised (memorised) 'cues' that alerted her to Ellen's deterioration in her usual state of health. Jane was consciously assessing Ellen's emotional and physical state of health as she sat with her. Some might call this the 'art of nursing' – being able to pick up cues in a given situation and make sense of what was possibly happening, make a clinical judgement and take appropriate action.

Professionally, 'being literate' means nurses need to look at how, and why, certain nursing interventions are planned, why we do and do not instigate care, and what factors influence our care decisions. In the past, nursing was 'taught' via word of mouth and by allowing trainees to watch and copy practice. Later on, nurses noted down core practice, and it was doctors and surgeons who wrote nursing textbooks based around their practice. Weir-Hughes (2010), Summers and Summers (2010) and Santry (2010) feel that if nurses write more about their practice, explaining why we nurse the way we do, this will enhance the image of nursing as a professional discipline in three ways, by

1. clarifying the role nurses play in participating and leading multidisciplinary teams;
2. demonstrating how we can not only act as patient advocates but also be advocates for health (working at more strategic and political levels to influence health and social care decisions);
3. showing how we can influence service improvement.

Nurses need, therefore, to be able to adopt different modes of communication to fit different needs. Being able to *write well is an essential element of good communication* (World, 2004).

Writing well: core principles

The Plain English Campaign (2010) believes that *everyone should have access to clear and concise information* (see box below). The need for 'plain' language is further endorsed within the NMC competencies (2.7).

Plain English Campaign's key points for effective writing (CPEC, 2010)

- Stop and think before you start writing. Make a note of the points you want to make in a logical order.
- Prefer short words.
- Use everyday English whenever possible. Avoid jargon and medical words, and always explain any technical terms you have to use.
- Keep your sentence length down to an average of 15 to 20 words. Try to stick to one main idea in a sentence.
- Use active verbs as much as possible. Say 'we will do it' rather than 'it will be done by us'.
- Be concise.
- Imagine you are talking to your reader. Write sincerely, personally, in a style that is suitable and with the right tone of voice.
- Always check that your writing is clear, helpful, human and polite.

Adapted from *How to Write in Plain English Guide* (www.plainenglish.co.uk)

'Writing well' means organising your thoughts and then conveying them in the most lucid and appropriate 'written' form to a certain audience. You need to tune into your audience (i.e. the reader), identify what information they need and their preferred mode of 'written' communication (words, pictures, symbols), decide what to say and how to say it so that others can 'read' it, reflect on it, understand it, appraise its value and consider using the information where appropriate. You will have to consider the style of writing, the language you use and how the information is presented to the reader, ensuring 'it says what you think it says'.

Fifteen steps to 'writing well'

1. Clarify the purpose of the 'written' material.
2. Identify what you, or others, already know.
3. Raise questions about what you, and or others, want to know.
4. Find relevant, valid, reliable and current information (the answers).
5. Summarise your findings around the priorities to be addressed.
6. Outline your response:
   (a) content; possible paragraphs of information;
   (b) how it is going to 'look', i.e. font, use of colour, diagrams or images, spacing.
7. Discuss your approach with a tutor, mentor, peer or patient group.
8. Do a draft by collating (bringing together) your notes in a logical order.
9. Get more feedback.
10. Review and edit the contents again . . . and again.
11. Write an introduction:
    (a) clearly stating the topic;
    (b) explaining how you have chosen to address the issue.
12. Write your conclusion:
    (a) restate the topic;
    (b) describe which particular aspects have been covered;
    (c) what you have learnt;
    (d) What has been left unanswered.
13. Do a spelling and grammar check 'by eye' as well as on the computer. (Computer spell check systems may not recognise some words, e.g. carer; or distinguish appropriate use of similar sounding words such as 'where', 'were' and 'wear'.)
14. Check your work is easy to read and legible, especially if handwritten. (A good way to check this is to read it out loud. If you stumble, consider rewriting sentences or checking grammar – see Temple, 2005.)
15. Finalise and submit your work.

You may need to repeat steps 8–10 several times. Therefore, scheduling your work is important. Your mentor or practice supervisor may need to authorise your work if, for example, it is a care plan or discharge letter. In patient information, as well as in your academic work, you must ensure your sources are referenced to avoid plagiarism (see Chapter 2, page 33). The word allowance will influence the final product – for example, a two-sided A4 patient information leaflet will require more precise and focused writing than a 3,500-word essay. The structure of the final written piece will vary depending on whether it's a care plan, report, letter or patient education leaflet (see Table 5.4 overleaf).

Care plan	Discharge letter or patient report	A clinical report leaflet	Patient education
• Assessments(s) • Aim • Expected outcomes of care (goals/objectives) • Planned interventions • Nursing record of care given • Evaluation of care	• Diagnosis • History of illness • Summary of medical, nursing and paramedical care • Arrangements for ongoing care • Patient's and/or carer's understanding of the situation • Further needs • Contacts for information or support	• Topic • Aim • Literature review • Methodology • Findings • Discussion • Recommendations for practice/further research • References • Appendices	• Health problem or illness • Explanation of cause, signs and symptoms • When to 'act' and seek medical advice • Investigations and procedures people commonly undergo • Common medical treatments • Commonly asked questions • Self-help • Contacts

Table 5.4: Structures for different written work

Documenting nursing assessments, care plans and writing nursing records

In completing your practice experience you will learn to write patient care plans and nursing records, complete referral forms and write discharge letters, and even participate in completion of court reports or patient education materials.

The ability to record the assessment, planning, implementation and evaluation of the effectiveness of care, and communicate care needs to others, is fundamental to protecting and maintaining high standards of integrated patient-centred care within multidisciplinary and multiagency settings (NMC, 2010a; Johnson et al., 2010; Lees, 2010; Law et al., 2010; NMC, 2009; Department of Health, 2007; Royal College of Nursing, 2005). Documentation of care often forms the basis of ward handovers and case conferences, and might be based on agreed 'care pathways'. Aims for care, expected patient outcomes and relevant planned interventions must be clear and open to regular review and evaluation at all stages of the patient experience.

Activity 5.2	*Critical thinking*

A senior nurse expressed her concern when nursing records contained comments such as 'care given as planned'.

Think of three reasons why writing 'care plan followed' or 'care given as planned' is insufficient.

An outline answer is provided at the end of the chapter.

In order to be accountable for your practice, it is important that not only patient's care needs are clearly and accurately recorded but that you also report on the outcome of the care provided, i.e. how effective measures were in relieving pain, how the potential development of pressure sores was managed, how well parents were able to provide a child's tracheostomy care before transfer home, how monitoring a clients' change in mood prevented self-harm. Remember you may be called to account for your care, professionally, in a court of law. When writing nursing records or reports ask yourself, frequently, if called to account for your practice tomorrow how well your nursing notes will reflect what took place yesterday.

Activity 5.3	*Leadership and management*

Imagine you have been asked to take part in an audit of nursing records in your hospital. List the criteria you would set to audit the quality of the documentation.

Review your list against the NMC (2010a) guidelines on writing patient documentation. You can access this document at **www.nmc-uk.org/Documents/Guidance/nmc GuidanceRecordKeepingGuidanceforNursesandMidwives.pdf**

There is a brief outline of criteria for good record-keeping at the end of the chapter. You might want to use your notes to assess your own practice.

Clinically, poor handwritten communication (illegible handwriting, poor spelling, incorrect terminology and incomplete documentation) has been reported as an underlying factor for misunderstanding patients' needs (Davies, 2010; Aiken and Dale, 2007), drug errors or omissions in care (NMC, 2010b; Luettal and Bischler, 2010; Krischke, 2009), mismatches between care being delivered and what is documented in care plans (Lees, 2010; Johnson et al., 2010), and even unnecessary readmission to hospital (Witherington et al., 2007). Lees's study, for example, found that information in nursing records was often unfocused or omitted, focused on that day's care rather than illustrating expected progress and future care, lacked evidence of systematic assessment and planning of care, that risk assessments were separate from care plans, and there was a lack of written evaluation of care evident. Her project identified eight elements to effective care planning and record-keeping. These included checklists for information needed on admission, selection of care plans appropriate to patient needs, developing a multi-disciplinary information sheet to be used for discharge planning, and a need for training of staff in how to write and evaluate care plans to ensure specific timely documentation of patient care.

Activity 5.4   *Reflection*

Look at a patient's nursing documentation that you participated in writing. Using the following, reflect on how well the written care plan documented:

(a) the patient's history; expected progress; actual care needed and/or previously given, and if any evaluation of care was undertaken;
(b) the aim of the patient's care;
(c) clear instructions for the care needed, the time frames for care to be given, and who was to provide the care (outcomes or objectives);
(d) whether the patient was involved in writing the care plan, or agreed to it.

Ask yourself, would someone else be able to follow it without any explanation or clarification from you?

As this is a personal reflection, there is no outline answer provided.

In order for you to hand over the patient's care to another nurse or healthcare professional, or write a referral or discharge letter, you need to ensure you clearly summarise the patient's experience, how their care needs have been met, and identify ongoing needs. It might be useful to write an action plan to develop your documentation skills in practice and discuss this with your mentor or practice supervisor. If you have concerns about the legibility of your handwriting there are some useful resources identified at the end of the chapter. You might find it useful to get someone to give you feedback on your handwriting. I know my students have often challenged me about being unable to read my handwritten comments on their assignments. I have learnt the reasons why my handwriting is not always clear could be related to the pen I use, how I sit to write, how I hold my pen, the speed I am writing, or whether I print or use joined–up (cursive) handwriting – to name but a few.

Care plans reflect the clinical decisions we make to provide appropriate care to patients. As such, they must be supported by accessible written protocols for care, policies and procedures (NMC, 2010a; Nottingham University Hospital, 2010). Such documents demonstrate how well we understand the rationale (grounds or reasons) for our practice; especially when there may be several ways to meet patient needs. The following case study highlights what can happen when we fail to work to current guidelines for good practice.

Case study

Rose, a 61-year-old single woman, was admitted for an elective left hip replacement for the treatment of osteoarthritis. She was asked to come to the ward at 7 a.m. ready for surgery, and ensure she had nothing to eat

continued opposite . . .

continued . . .

or drink from 12 midnight the previous day. Rose was orientated onto the ward and prepared for her surgery. She eventually went to theatre at 3.30 p.m. that day. Her care plan indicated for her to remain nil by mouth until her surgery.

Activity 5.5   *Critical thinking and evidence-based practice*

Read the case study and then consider the following.

* How well do you think the instructions given to Rose pre-operatively met her fluid and nutritional needs prior to her surgery?
* Did they reflect current guidelines for 'starving' patients prior to surgery?
* How would you rewrite the nursing care instructions to maintain her nutritional needs and fluid balance pre- and post-operatively?
* Why do you think the nurses were not working to current guidelines for pre-operative starving?

An outline answer is provided at the end of the chapter.

On practice learning experience you will see that a patient in hospital may have a number of documents by their bed, such as:

* admission self-assessment
* observation chart
* mobility assessment
* nutritional assessment
* care plan
* pre-op check list
* drug chart.

All these documents require completion in handwriting. The clarity can vary according to each nurse's handwriting style. There may be no summary of how these documents have been used in planning, giving and evaluating care shift by shift. This means that the nurse receiving handover would have had to sift through each document to make sense of the patient's current care needs. Think about the patient documentation you have come across. You too will have to make sense of and collate a variety of information, and subsequently write detailed information, succinctly and clearly to reflect your participation, and others', in patient care.

Writing for clients (improving health literacy)

As a nursing student you might find yourself writing down information for patients (to support verbal instruction) and/or take part in producing patient information.

Health literacy is defined as *the intellectual and social capacity to make informed decisions on health matters* (Hubley and Copeman, 2008, p27). In plain language this means that people need to be able to find, 'read', understand and use health information where appropriate to take action to maintain or improve their health, or cope with long-term illness. Printed media, leaflets and posters are one source of health information that the Department of Health and NHS rely on to inform people about risks to their health; how their health may be influenced by their own lifestyle choices; and/or how their work and/or the environment might influence their health.

Not all of this information is supported by alternative media such as audio recordings and videos. This means that, as healthcare professionals, we are often reliant on people's ability to read and understand written literature in making health choices. In addition, you will have to help people who have been bombarded and worried by 'scary' information in television advertisements or on the internet, not all of which is always appropriate or effective. In order to make informed decisions about stopping smoking, or being immunised, for example, people will rely on the information you give them verbally and/or in the form of patient education leaflets. Unfortunately, many people have low reading ability (Department of Education, 2010). Low health literacy has been associated with poor communication between patients and healthcare providers, increased hospitalisation rates, less frequent utilisation of screening and immunisation services, inappropriate use of accident and emergency services instead of primary healthcare services to manage minor illness, and inability to understand how to take or use medication (White et al., 2010; Easton et al., 2010; Shaw et al., 2009; Protheroe et al., 2009; Wagner et al., 2009).

The NMC competencies require you to assess patients' needs for health information and provide relevant information to clients to improve their health. You will need to:

- familiarise yourself with the patient information that is current;
- assess its reliability and credibility before you recommend it to patients (just as you would for any information used to inform your nursing practice);
- adapt your use of 'written' forms of communication with the patient, and/or their carers, to meet their level of literacy;
- design and develop appropriate health promotion materials such as health promotion posters and patient information leaflets.

Activity 5.6   *Communication*

Pick up a leaflet in your GP practice, or an outpatients clinic, that is relevant to your own health needs. It could be related to immunisation, screening, understanding medication, or explaining a potential or actual illness or treatment.

Use the following eight criteria to assess how well it meets your needs.
1. Who is the leaflet aimed at (target group)?
2. Is the information relevant to you? If so, why; if not, why?
3. How credible is the author?
4. Is there any hidden agenda, i.e. advertising of a product through sponsorship of the leaflet?
5. Is the information up to date (current)?
6. Is the information easy to read and understand?

continued opposite . . .

continued . . . .

7. Did it leave with you with any questions unanswered, and, if so
8. Were any contacts identified for more information or support?

(Adapted from Ewles and Simnet, 2003; Department of Health, 2003)

As this is based on individual research, there is no outline answer provided.

Health information tends to be aimed at the general population. It doesn't always meet specific patient needs, i.e. reflect age, gender or social and cultural circumstances (race, ethnicity, language, nationality, religion, sexual orientation, income level and occupation). The information may also challenge accepted attitudes, values and 'normal' patterns of behaviour – for example, men and women may have different needs for information. Women from different communities may need the information given in different ways. For example, you might want to encourage breast self-awareness in women generally, but some of the recommended health actions may be a cause of embarrassment for Muslim women. In addition, women with learning disabilities might need a more pictorial form of information to understand how to be 'breast aware' (see Willis et al., 2008). It is also worth noting that although there is a small incidence of breast cancer in men there is no information specifically directed at men on being 'breast aware'. One of the men in the cancer support group I work with suggested that perhaps men would react more favourably to information about 'breast awareness' if it was called 'chest awareness' (and not always in pink).

The Department of Health, Robinson (2003), Hubley and Copeman (2008), and Ewles and Simnet (2003) offer useful pointers for writing patient information. These are summarised in Table 5.5 overleaf.

Activity 5.7   *Reflection*

Reflect on a patient you have recently nursed in relation to how you:

*   assessed their need for information;
*   decided what information was appropriate;
*   provided the information, particularly if written;
*   assessed the patient's understanding of and likelihood they could act on the information;
*   recorded the activity in your nursing notes.

As this is a personal exercise, there is no outline answer provided.

Many nurses have difficulty in identifying their health promotion role. However, this could be resolved easily if our nursing documentation reflected how we:

*   assessed patient understanding of their health and/or illness;
*   managed their care needs to prevent problems, detect problems early and resolve them, or assisted them in the management of long-term problems;
*   recorded the supportive information as given to patients and monitored their understanding (e.g. patient information prescriptions);
*   identified who we involved, why and how in the delivery of care.

The message	The format	Design with the user	Use with the patient
Main message on the front.	Use simple language.	Find out what patients want* to know.	Use 'teach-back' to ensure the patient's understanding:
Consider cultural differences.	Define technical terms.	Add what they need* to know.	1. Patient 'reads'.
No more than four points.	Use short words and sentences (line length 40–50 characters; 15–20 words a sentence).	Verify information with relevant professional bodies.	2. Ask them to restate the information in their own words.
Focus on the action or behaviour needed, e.g. take your medication at 10.00 in the morning every day.	Avoid jargon, abbreviations and clichés.	Explore what will help reading/use of the information.	3. Repeat the information and feedback until both happy.
Keep it short and specific.	Use headings to break up the text.	Ask patients to pre-test the information.	Enhance patient's understanding by asking them 'to write' the information down in their own words (if able).
Ensure step-by-step instructions, where appropriate, with explanations.	Use captions or cues to highlight key information.	Do a readability test.	
Signpost other services, resources and support.	Use **bold** to highlight points.	* what patients want and need to know may be different	
Read it aloud; if you can't – rewrite.	Use simple line drawings.		
	Number lists rather than use bullet points.		
	Use 12-point font sans serif.		
	Avoid use of all capitals.		
	Leave plenty of white space.		
	Choose colours with care.		
	Include universal symbols and clear signage.		

Table 5.5: Key tips for creating patient information

Most pre-registration programmes ask student nurses to maintain a portfolio to reflect their learning. Self-assessment, peer assessment, mentor and even patient assessment documentation could be used to demonstrate your developing professional expertise in writing a variety of nursing documentation, over time, through different clinical experiences. In addition, as a professional nurse, you need to write about and share your current practice and be prepared to offer your practice up to the scrutiny of others. This is often referred to as 'scholarly activity'. Once you are a registered practitioner, you will need to develop these skills further in order to make authoritative recommendations for practice – for example, to write nursing procedures and policy, publish in academic journals and/or present papers at conferences.

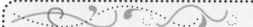

Chapter summary

Writing well is an important part of 'being literate' as a nurse. It can take different forms. It is apparent that assessment of literacy is more than assessing an individual nurse's ability to read, write and use written professional documentation. It is more holistic: it's about how we package (assess, plan, implement and evaluate care) and ultimately document the finite distinctions of what makes effective nursing practice.

Activities: Brief outline answers

Activity 5.2 (page 103)

Writing 'Care given as planned' is insufficient in nursing records because the reader is:

- unable to assess effectiveness or appropriateness of care;
- has difficulty seeing continuity of care maintained;
- has difficulty seeing if the person who planned the care was the person who gave or supervised the care, making it difficult to see who was accountable for care;
- has difficulty seeing patient satisfaction or involvement with care.

Activity 5.3 (page 103)

You may have included some or all of the following.

- Correct terminology used.
- Language used is common, authorised, across all professionals.
- Abbreviations approved by trust.
- Written clearly, in ink, legible.
- In chronological order.
- Signed and printed name and status; where necessary countersigned.
- Time and date included.
- Corrections:
    (a) cross out with a single line;
    (b) indicate 'written in error';
    (c) date and sign the correction.

Activity 5.5 (page 105)

Maintaining someone's hydration and nutrition is an essential part of any patient's hospital stay (NMC, 2007, 2008b, 2010c). The essence of care guidelines 'Agreed person-focused outcome' is that *People are enabled to consume food and drink (orally) which meets their needs and preferences* (Department of Health, 2010, p7). Current guidelines around pre-operative starving advise that patients can have clear oral fluids up to two hours before surgery, and a light diet up to six hours prior to surgery (**www.surgical-tutor.org.uk**). Rose's care needs were not reassessed once the nurses knew she was on the afternoon surgery list. In doing so there was a potential clinical risk of dehydration and electrolyte disturbance, and Rose was left unnecessarily thirsty and hungry, which could have added to her discomfort prior to her surgery. Revising her care plan, plus writing on the 'notice board' above her bed, what and when she could eat and drink, would have ensured her diet and fluids were appropriate prior to her surgery.

Aim of her care plan: to maintain her normal fluid and fluid intake by alternative means while being nil by mouth prior to surgery.

Intervention: Rose can have a light diet until 10 a.m. and clear fluids until 1 p.m.

Nurses may not have adjusted her care plan because they were not aware of the guidelines, were reluctant to challenge routine care which dictated patients be starved from 12 midnight, or were not prepared to be accountable for altering the planned care.

Further reading

Austin, S (2006) Ladies & gentlemen of the jury, I present . . . the nursing documentation. *Nursing,* January, 36 (1): 56–63.

This article provides a neat introduction about why documentation is important when faced with a coroner. References and further reading may be available for this article. To view these you must purchase the article.

Department of Health (2003) *Toolkit for producing patient information, version 2.* London: Department of Health.

Department of Health (2004) *Good practice in patient care and improving the patient experience: patient information leaflets and comment cards.* London: Department of Health.

Both of the above provide an essential guide to producing effective, clear and accessible patient information.

Lees, L (2010) Improving the quality of nursing documentation on an acute medicine unit. *Nursing Times,* 106 (37): 22–26, 21 September.

Identifies some of the factors that influence good patient documentation.

NMC (2010) *Guidelines for records and record keeping. Guidance for Nurses and Midwives.* London: NMC.

Essential reading to underpin good practice.

Temple, M (2005) *Grammar Book.* Oxford: Blackwell.

One of the best guides to grammar, which helps remind you of the essentials.

Useful websites

www.ehow.com/how_5464189_improve-handwriting.html

This web page has some useful tips on effective penmanship. If you are often told that people cannot read your handwriting it may be worth a look.

www.nmc-uk.org/http://www.nmc-uk.org/Documents/Guidance/

nmcGuidanceRecordKeepingGuidanceforNursesandMidwives.pdf

An essential document to underpin your record-keeping.

www.plainenglish.co.uk

The Plain English website provides a useful background on how to write in a format that is accessible to anyone. It has some useful examples and resources.

Chapter 6
Technology skills: making the computer work for you

Karen Sumpton

NMC Standards for Pre-registration Nursing Education

This chapter will address the following competencies:

Domain 1: Professional values

7. All nurses must be responsible and accountable for keeping their knowledge and skills up to date through continuing professional development. They must aim to improve their performance and enhance the safety and quality of care through evaluation, supervision and appraisal.

Domain 2: Communication and interpersonal skills

2. All nurses must use a range of communication skills and technologies to support person-centred care and enhance quality and safety. They must ensure people receive all the information they need in a language and manner that allows them to make informed choices and share decision-making. They must recognise when language interpretation or other communication support is needed and know how to obtain it.

Domain 3: Nursing practice and decision-making

1. All nurses must use up-to-date knowledge and evidence to assess, plan, deliver and evaluate care, communicate findings, influence change and promote health and best practice. They must make person-centred, evidence-based judgments and decisions, in partnership with others involved in the care process, to ensure high quality care. They must be able to recognise when the complexity of clinical decisions requires specialist knowledge and expertise, and consult or refer accordingly.

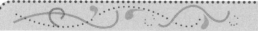

NMC Essential Skills Clusters

This chapter will address the following ESCs:

Cluster: Care, compassion and communication

1. As partners in the care process, people can trust a newly registered graduate nurse to provide collaborative care based on the highest standards, knowledge and competence.

continued overleaf . . .

continued . . . •••

By the first progression point:

1. Articulates the underpinning values of *The Code: Standards of conduct, performance and ethics for nurses and midwives* (the *Code*) (NMC, 2008b).
2. Works within limitations of the role and recognises own level of competence.
3. Promotes a professional image.
4. Shows respect for others.

Cluster: Medicines management

39. People can trust a newly registered graduate nurse to keep and maintain accurate records using information technology, where appropriate, within a multi-disciplinary framework as a leader and as part of a team and in a variety of care settings including at home.

Chapter aims

By the end of this chapter, you should be able to:

- identify the main ICT skills expected of nursing students;
- be aware of the two main ICT qualifications to prove competence;
- describe the main Web 2.0 tools and apply their use in both an educational setting and in clinical practice;
- list the advantages and possible uses of mobile technologies in clinical practice.

Introduction

If you are undertaking your nursing training later in life, perhaps after having children, you may be wondering how much information technology (IT) knowledge you will need in your role. Even if you started your training at an earlier age, you may not be familiar with all the IT you will be introduced to throughout your programme. The field of IT moves quickly, and new technologies are being introduced all the time. These new technologies need not be daunting if you are aware that they exist and can build up your confidence in using them. This chapter introduces IT software and technologies that you will find useful as a practising nurse.

In recent years, nursing education, in common with general higher education trends, has changed for several reasons. First, the nursing student population has changed and comprises both young people who have been brought up in the digital age (sometimes called 'digital natives') and who embrace technology such as computers, the Internet, and mobile phones and use them to their full advantage, and those students who may be non-traditional learners, the so-called 'digital immigrants,' who were born before the digital age but have adopted it to some extent. There has also been an increase in the number of nursing students in employment who study part-time, and in the numbers who elect to study at a distance. Within the Health Service, practitioners are increasingly working alone, often practising in more remote areas where access to information, support and other resources is limited. This trend is set to increase further as the focus on care continues to move into the community (Longley, 2007).

Technology is changing at a rapid rate. Emerging technologies now provide highly interactive, collaborative and reflective learning environments, which foster communication and enable immediate access to knowledge. Information and Communications Technology (ICT) has enabled learning and knowledge sharing to take place outside the confines of the classroom and has resulted in different delivery modes, such as electronic learning (e-learning), whereby students can learn within a virtual environment at their convenience. Traditional learning methods are therefore less likely to attract students and maintain attention and engagement. Those studying at a distance need access to information and a support network to prevent feelings of isolation, and technology can make this happen. For you as a nursing student, learning how to use these technologies effectively at an early stage will help not only during your studies, but also in the future when in clinical practice, particularly in terms of your continuing professional development.

In this chapter we will look at the skills you need not only in your studies, but also in clinical practice. You are provided with information about what these skills are and when you might want to use them. Learning does not stop when you finish your course – it should be a lifelong experience – and these skills provide you with the opportunity to access information and knowledge wherever you are based.

Activity 6.1   *Reflection*

This activity will encourage you to reflect on how confident you feel about your own ICT skills.

- Use a search engine to find the full definition of the terms 'digital native' and 'digital immigrant'.
- Consider your own ICT skills. Are you a digital native or immigrant?

There is no right or wrong answer to the activity and even if you feel hesitant about using computers, realising this and continuing through this chapter will help you to recognise the value of acquiring or brushing up on those skills.

As this is based on your own skills development, there is no outline answer provided.

ICT skills

If you are perhaps returning to education or consider yourself to be a digital immigrant, it is possible that you do not have much experience of working with computers. In this case, in order to be able to cope with the standard of work expected of you both during your course and afterwards in clinical practice, learning about computers and the main software applications is essential.

Even if you class yourself as a digital native, are a regular user of software such as Word, Excel, etc., and regard yourself as competent in these areas, it is likely that you are self-taught. As such, you may not know all of the software features that can make life much easier and enable you to produce work of a high standard. It may therefore help you to brush up on those skills and to prove your competence by obtaining a recognised qualification.

Basic skills and file management

If you are new to computers, they can be pretty daunting initially. The hardest part is getting started as there seems so much to learn and some people fear making mistakes or breaking something. Understanding the basics of your computer is important as it can help you to use it efficiently and keep it functioning well.

Organising your files will enable you to find them again later. As your studies progress and you create more documents and other files, you will find it increasingly difficult to find what you are looking for as you search through possibly hundreds of filenames; people tend to hoard files rather than deleting those they no longer need. The ability to create folders, move files into those folders, and to delete files and folders might seem basic, but it is important. Understanding how to save your work properly, how to back up your files, and how to work between different software versions is vital so that you do not lose any of your work.

Word processing

Possibly the most widely used of the Microsoft Office applications is Word, which is used for word processing documents such as reports and assignments. Some people simply use the software to type up their work but never fully utilise all of Word's features, features that could make life easier and enable you to produce work to a professional standard. For example, when preparing a long document, you could make use of Word's headers and footers to include additional information, such as chapter headings, page numbering, or your name and unique student number repeated on every page. Another way of enhancing your document would be to include images, which can often be found on the Internet. You can save those images and then insert them into your assignment to illustrate a point. Word allows you to move, resize or crop images, or to add picture styles to further improve the look of your document.

You can also create your own diagrams using Word's Autoshapes, or if using one of the later versions (2007 or 2010) you could use the SmartArt feature, which contains a variety of different layouts from which to choose. Acquiring Word skills will enable you to group images and shapes together to create one 'object' which can be easily moved, and you could use text boxes to add labels. For example, you might wish to create an organisation chart in a report document after attending a course. In SmartArt, you are provided with a skeleton structure of the chart, which you can then complete with specific information, saving you time in creating your own chart from scratch.

Word contains a list of styles – pre-set formatting for text. These are particularly useful for formatting headings and subheadings consistently throughout your document, and they are easy to apply and modify. If you format your main headings in capitals, for example, then all main headings will be in capitals, which makes it easier for your reader to follow. Have you ever tried to create your own table of contents? If you create a table of contents by typing it

Contents

1 Introduction 1
2 What is punishment? 1
3 What is Just Punishment? 2
  3.1 Theory 3
4 Justified Retributive Theory 4
  4.1 Generalisation 5
5 Justifying Punishment 6
  5.1 Communication..7
6 Problems 8
7 Alternatives 9
  7.1 Morality 10
8 Conclusion 11
9 Bibliography 12

Figure 6.1: Formatting for a table of contents

into your document it can be hard to line up the page numbers, particularly if you want to set it out as in Figure 6.1, using dots (tab leaders) after the title, then right-aligning the page numbers.

If you do it all by hand, then if you later need to move sections around, you have to check the new page numbers and retype them, which can be tedious. If you use styles for all your headings, Word can easily create an automatic table of contents, table of figures and table of tables, which will be perfectly aligned, have the correct page numbers, and can be updated with a couple of clicks.

Spreadsheets

Excel is a Microsoft spreadsheet application. You might think that spreadsheets will not be of use to you, but they are extremely useful for organising and analysing data. Often during your studies, you will be required to collect data from various sources, such as questionnaires. Effective use of Excel enables you to display the data in a logical manner and offers the opportunity to display the data graphically using charts, make calculations and find trends, thus making your document more interesting and much more readable. You can then easily import such information into a Word document to support your findings or illustrate a point you have made. Report writing in clinical practice is frequent, and the ability to properly analyse and present data in your document is important.

Activity 6.2 — *Critical thinking*

Helen is a practice nurse and is monitoring the weight loss of a group of patients who have recently given birth. The two images overleaf represent the same set of data. Which do you think looks best and why?

Which image is easier to understand?

continued overleaf . . .

Image 1:

Weight loss (pounds)						
	January	February	March	April	May	June
Jane	9	6	5	6	4	7
Abigail	12	8	6	7	5	4
Linda	8	9	7	6	7	5
Claire	14	8	6	4	5	6

Image 2:

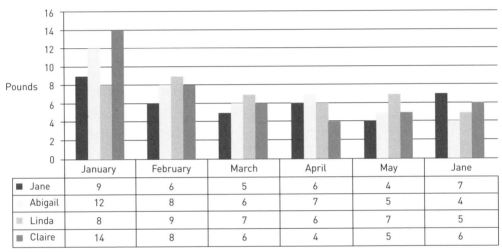

An outline answer is provided at the end of the chapter.

Databases

A database is simply an organised collection of data. Microsoft Access is a widely used **database application** and enables you to store information in tables, **interrogate** the data by asking questions of it using Queries, and produce reports. Databases are very similar to spreadsheets but they offer you more flexibility and are much more powerful at manipulating data.

As a nursing student, when looking for information you will be using databases. They are just like an Access database in that they store information, in this case journal articles. You can also create your own databases. Some can be simply recreational, such as organising your DVD collection; others could be for professional reasons, such as setting up a database containing contact details of Health Trusts etc. to which you might apply for jobs in the future. Nurses running travel immunisation clinics need databases of every country's requirement for travellers, the source of each treatment, costs and so on. Being able to create a **mail merge** using Word and pulling in address information from a database makes the task easier than writing to each Trust individually, and it enables you to keep track of the tasks you have completed so far so that you do not duplicate work.

Presentations

As a nursing student, presenting your work will be part of your course. A presentation should only list brief points, which you can then explain in full, and it should engage the audience. Microsoft Office contains a presentation package called PowerPoint, which enables you to create a professional-looking presentation quickly and easily. You can use on-screen slides to represent each point you make. You can change the layout of slides to fit the information you have – for example, provide a bulleted list or two-column text. PowerPoint contains a host of designs and themes that enable you to add colour and interest to both your text and backgrounds. You can also incorporate slide transitions (the way that the presentation moves from one slide to the next – for example, fade in from the top), and you can animate both text and images. You can also import data from Excel into your presentation, creating dynamic links so that your presentation will automatically update if you change data in your Excel file. These are very useful skills to acquire now, while you are a student. When you are nursing, you will often present information to interprofessional team members.

Case study

Sue is a practice nurse and has just returned from a two-day course on COPD. She needs to disseminate all the material to her colleagues at a meeting tomorrow. Luckily, she learned as a student how to put together a PowerPoint presentation, and put all the data from the course onto her laptop. Sue was able to read through her notes and then quickly create a professional-looking presentation that she then delivered to her colleagues. She provided a copy of the presentation on the Intranet so they could refer back to it when necessary.

Email

Communication is no longer just face to face, by letter or by telephone. The ability to contact someone at any time has huge advantages in that they don't actually have to be there at the time that you send the message. Email enables the message to sit in their inbox until that person is free to send you a response. There is also a written record of the communication, to which it is useful to refer back.

There are many email packages available, many of which are Internet-based, such as Hotmail, Yahoo Mail, etc. Microsoft Office contains the Outlook application, which is widely used outside colleges and universities and so is useful to learn for employability. Outlook is not just about email; it also contains features such as a calendar, contacts, tasks and notes, and is therefore useful for organising yourself.

Email is often regarded as conversational and therefore informal rather than formal. Whichever email package you use, there are informal rules of etiquette that you should follow when communicating.

- **To email or not to email?** Before writing an email, consider whether you really need to send one at all. Would it be better to go and see the person face to face or pick up the phone and speak to them direct?
- **Subject**: Always include a subject line as this gives the recipient a clue as to the content.
- **Confidentiality**: If your message is confidential, make that clear at the start. Outlook has the capability to mark an email as confidential.
- **External communication**: Not everyone uses the same email software as you; therefore, if there is doubt, it is preferable to send your message using Rich Text or Plain Text as HTML may make your email unreadable for some people.
- **Readability**: Shorter paragraphs and good use of white space make your message easier to read. Long reams of uninterrupted text may be off-putting to the recipient and encourage them to avoid reading your message.
- **Tone**: It is very difficult to ascertain the tone in a written email, which can lead to misunderstandings. Try not to be ambiguous and keep your tone professional. Do not use CAPITALS as it looks like shouting.
- **Attachments**: Try to avoid sending long attachments and keep them below 5Mb where possible. An alternative to emailing a large file might be to provide access to it via a website or the intranet, then to send a hyperlink to the document. Compressing (or 'zipping') files before attaching is another alternative, as this will reduce them in size.
- **Signatures**: It is good practice to include a signature in your email as this will provide the recipient with your credentials and give them easy access to your contact information for future reference.
- **Forwarding emails**: Think carefully before forwarding an incoming email. Is the message confidential? If you go ahead with forwarding the email, the original message is usually included. Take care to check the content before sending, as it might be advisable to delete anything of a personal nature or anything not strictly relevant.

Email is not a secure medium, therefore you need to take care about the information you include. For example, sending password information in an email is never appropriate. If it essential to let someone know a password, do it in person. Take care when writing with reference to someone else, since you cannot be sure that the recipient will not pass that information on to a third party, or worse, to the individual concerned.

In terms of incoming email, always view attachments with suspicion. If you do not know the sender, never open an attached file as this could transmit a virus to your computer. Beware of spoof emails that purport to come from a source you recognise. If in doubt, telephone the person concerned to check that they did send you the email. In clinical practice, it is important that any email communication with a patient is treated with the same gravity as a formal letter and you need to pay particular attention to your choice of wording and tone. Privacy must also be respected since emails can be intercepted or viewed easily, and copies must be kept in the patient's records.

Learning how to use these software packages properly makes life easier for you and prepares you for your professional future, transforming you into an individual who confidently uses ICT skills, which, in turn, support lifelong learning.

Recognised qualifications

European Computer Driving Licence

The European Computer Driving Licence (ECDL) is a nationally recognised qualification that enables you to develop your skills in the use of computers and obtain proof of your competence. It requires no previous knowledge of computers and is not restricted to any specific software package. ECDL comprises seven units.

- IT security for users
- IT user fundamentals
- Word processing
- Spreadsheets
- Databases
- Presentations
- Using email and the Internet

You must pass all seven tests in order to complete the qualification. Acquiring certification in ECDL not only proves your competence level in these areas, but also enables you to work confidently with applications to produce work of a high standard.

Essential IT Skills qualification

An alternative to ECDL is Essential IT Skills (EITS), which focuses on the delivery of two qualifications: NHS Elite and NHS Health. Both qualifications are accredited by the British Computer Society and are mapped to the NHS Knowledge and Skills Framework (KSF). Training is delivered in a variety of ways: classroom-based via an NHS training department, online, via CD-Rom, via a Learning Management System (LMS), or by paper-based materials.

There are three practical tests for the NHS Elite qualification and content covers basic IT skills such as how to use a mouse and keyboard through to file management, web and email skills. The NHS Health qualification comprises just one practical test. This programme is aimed at candidates who come into contact with health systems in their job roles. As well as some basic IT skills, participants learn about patient confidentiality, accessing patient records, retrieval of information, navigating and documenting personal data.

Web 2.0 and emerging technologies

Having looked at the main ICT skills you will need, we now turn to recent and emerging technologies, which are becoming more and more widely used. Emerging technologies, such as

Web 2.0 tools (pronounced 'Web two oh'), have allowed education and knowledge sharing to move outside the confines of the classroom. The Internet not only allows access to a wealth of information, but also provides opportunities for non-traditional educational providers, such as virtual colleges, and supports the lifelong learning needs of practitioners, no matter where they are based.

Web 2.0 is a term associated with Web content that is generated by people using the Web. Content could be a photograph, a video, a list of Web links or a personal profile, and is placed on the Web by anyone using the Web to be accessible to other Web users. Web 2.0 tools make learning more interactive and focus on communication and collaboration, connecting geographically dispersed people with others working in the same field, thus facilitating the sharing of ideas and experience and giving the opportunity to provide mutual support. In effect, you work within a virtual community, building relationships, sharing and evolving ideas, and all in real time. You therefore learn from your social network in a community of practice.

Web 2.0 tools include:

- social networking sites, such as Facebook, MySpace, Bebo, and Ning;
- blogs and microblogs, such as Twitter;
- wikis, such as Wikipedia;
- video-sharing sites, such as YouTube.

Social networking

Due to the collaborative nature of Web 2.0 tools, many equate them with the term 'social software'. Social networks share certain characteristics. When you create an account, they tend to provide you with a profile page where you can put as much or as little information as you wish. The most important characteristic is the ability to find friends, those you have lost touch with, those you already know, and to make new friends. You can therefore build a network of friends, or a social network. Examples of social networks are Facebook, MySpace and Bebo.

Although people, particularly teenagers, use social networking sites to contact friends, these sites can also be used to connect with a network of fellow professionals. Users can join groups formed around common interests or goals. Such a network group is important for employment opportunities, sharing practice and creating research partnerships. As a nursing student, using social networking sites such as Facebook to keep in contact with friends and family is fine, but you should consider widening your professional network by checking for appropriate groups to join through the site. There you can make friends with others who are either studying or working in your profession. You can share ideas and provide support for each other and build relationships that you will take into the future.

Social networking sites specifically for health professionals include ProNurse and NurseLinkUp. Other networking sites such as LinkedIn have health professionals networks available. The Royal College of Nursing's website explains more about social networking and provides links to some networking sites you might want to investigate. Social networking can be very useful in providing you with information about what is going on in your profession and allowing you to learn from the experience of others, as well as passing on your thoughts and ideas. However, be aware that whatever you write can be viewed by others. Letting off steam if you are feeling under pressure or aggrieved about something can cause you problems, possibly of a disciplinary nature. Think twice before you have a rant or at the very least you will seem unprofessional. The NMC also require you to conduct yourself personally and professionally as specified in the NMC *Guidance on Professional Conduct for Nursing and Midwifery Students* (2010d), and this sets out specific requirements related to social networking.

> *Abide by UK laws and the rules, regulation, policies and procedures of the university and clinical placement providers with regard to your use of the internet and social networking sites.*

> *Ensure that you are familiar with and follow our advice on the use of social networking sites (available from our website www.nmc-uk.org).*

Also, be careful about what personal information you give away. No matter what your reasons are for using social networking sites, you should never let people know your address, phone number or date of birth as this might invite unwelcome attention or even identity fraud. Never give out any financial information, or worse, bank details. Be careful about any personal information you display, who you speak to and what you say, so that it doesn't come back to haunt you. Remember, colleagues and senior staff can access information, and so can patients and their relatives. It is essential that you abide by the NMC *Code* of conduct and therefore do not present yourself to the world with photographs or words of an unsavoury nature. Finally, confidentiality is vital, therefore never gossip about patients or colleagues.

Blogs

A blog (short for weblog) is a format for publishing content on the Web. Blogs are usually an online journal or diary, set up by people who invite comments and discussion from others. Blogs usually have the following features in common.

- The content is arranged in reverse chronological order so that the most recent entry is at the top of the Web page.
- Each entry has a date and time stamp.
- The blog software usually automatically generates archives to form a historical repository.

In an educational context, a blog can be created and used by an online group of students who have a shared interest. One such blog was established at Montgomery College, USA, and was used by a study group in the Faculty of Nursing. A face-to-face orientation session was held to help first-time users familiarise themselves both with each other and with posting comments on the blog. The online icebreaker helped individuals to feel part of the group and they became enthused by this new, dynamic, real-time method of communication. Thereafter, online discussions took place outside the classroom, involving such topics as the readings and activities set by the tutors (Shaffer et al., 2006). It was found that the students' learning experience at Montgomery was enhanced by the opportunity to share their thoughts and ideas, to ask questions in a non-threatening environment, and use the Internet as a valuable resource tool, supplying each other with links to other sites. As well as increasing their online collaborative skills, the students gained by feeling very much part of the virtual community where mutual support was at the forefront.

Twitter is a microblogging site that uses short messages called tweets (140 characters or less). Tweets can be sent via the Twitter website or through smart phones and are essentially a public conversation (Phillippi, 2010). The Royal College of Nursing has a Twitter page. You can register with Twitter and then search for any groups or institutions that you might find useful. Then simply choose to 'follow' them, and you will have access to any snippets of news and current information and advice.

Some people set up blogs for purely personal reasons, such as to write a journal while they are on holiday or travelling for pleasure, but a professional blog could be provided during your studies and it is worthwhile contributing to it as you can gain such a lot in terms of knowledge sharing and support. Setting up your own blog is easy. Hosted blogs allow you to sign up for an account and create a free blog. Such hosts include Blogger, Wordpress and Vox. All you have to do is choose a suitable name for the blog and then write some content. There are usually free tutorials on the provider's site, so look for those if you need help setting your blog up.

Activity 6.3   *Critical thinking*

- Use a search engine to search for blogs in your field. Name two of them that you might find useful to explore further. **Bookmark** them so that you can revisit them at your leisure.
- Go to the Royal College of Nursing blog page for students at **www.thercnstudent-bus.blogspot.com**. Do you think this blog is useful to student nurses?
- Reflect and think about why nursing students might find blogs useful.
- What problems might you encounter in using blogs as a learning resource?

An outline answer is provided at the end of the chapter.

Wikis

A wiki is a type of website that allows users to add, remove and edit content that can be quickly published to the Web. You do not need any knowledge of HTML programming language, which means that a wiki is an effective tool for collaboration as it is easy to use. Wikis allow knowledge to be quickly disseminated to the online community. There are open wikis to which anyone can contribute, and closed wikis that are set up for specific groups and are accessible only by password.

General wikis include Wikipedia, which is an online encyclopaedia that was created collaboratively and can be edited by anyone who wishes. Much of the information it contains is conceded to be authoritative (Younger, 2010), and at the very least it provides a good starting point with links to other sites of interest. Wikipedia is very useful for general information and can also act as a signpost to more professionally produced websites. Subject-specific wikis aimed at health professions including NursingWiki 2010, AskDrWiki, Medpedia and ganfyd. Medical and health wikis tend to be provided by specialist practitioners and are therefore authoritative. They provide information on medical conditions, drugs and medical procedures.

In an educational context, a wiki could be used for dissemination of information, providing access to documents and for sharing knowledge and experience among the group. Resources such as wikis should always be assessed against such criteria as who the authors are, the authors' credentials, how up to date the information is, and the range and quality of other resources it links to. Beware of using such sites as references in work submitted for assessment as they may not have the required credibility for useable evidence in your subject. Check your university's policies on this. (See also Chapter 8 for more on evaluating sources of evidence.) You can also set up your own wiki. Websites such as WikiSpaces or WetPaint allow you to create an account and set up a wiki, often free of charge.

Activity 6.4   *Critical thinking*

Using a search engine, find the ganfyd site and look up diabetes or any medical condition of your choice.

- Compare it with the same entry on Medpedia.
- Which provides you with more information?
- Which site do you prefer and why?

Some ideas concerning this activity are provided at the end of the chapter.

Media sharing

Media sharing allows users to upload and store photographs and videos on a central website. Other users can then access these resources. People can also join groups of others with a shared interest and contribute to a discussion board, sharing thoughts and ideas.

Photographs were the first form of media sharing. One of the earliest and most popular digital photo-sharing sites is Flickr, which allows you to upload photographs from a PC, phone or by email. You can also manipulate your photographs on Flickr, resizing, cropping, adjusting exposure and adding effects. Other well-known sites include Webshots and Photobucket. Video came later, with the most famous site being YouTube. This site offers a free online streaming service that allows anyone to view and share videos uploaded by registered users. You can search for virtually any subject and you will probably find it. Once you have chosen a video, YouTube will suggest related ones.

Videojug is a really good site providing 'how to' videos. It contains thousands of categorised videos, or there is a search feature you can use. You can even join the Videojug Facebook page or follow them on Twitter.

RSS feeds

RSS stands for 'Really Simple Syndication', sometimes referred to as Web feeds or just feeds. You may regularly check various web pages for current information – for example, The Nursing and Midwifery Council website, *The Nursing Times*, the Royal College of Nursing, etc. On many of the web pages you visit, you will see a link that looks like this 🔊 or RSS or may simply say 'Subscribe'. Clicking the link enables you to subscribe to that page so that in future you can view all your subscriptions in one place, instead of having to visit each individual page.

RSS feeds could include news headlines, links to your favourite journals, blogs, audio and video links. They are very similar to magazine subscriptions in that you don't have to keep going to the newsagent to get the latest information from your favourite magazines; you can sit back and wait for the new information to come to you.

RSS Aggregators take the RSS feed and convert it into readable, formatted content. Aggregators also check for new updated content and deliver it to you. Internet Explorer and Firefox can be used to subscribe to RSS feeds and read them directly in the browser, but you need to use the same PC to access those feeds in future. There are also several Web-based aggregators where you can create an account and have your feeds delivered to the online account. You can therefore access your feeds from anywhere that you have Internet access. Google Reader is an aggregator that is easy to use. It regularly checks your favourite news sites, blogs etc. for updates. You can even use the built-in public page to share items with friends and family. Other aggregators include Bloglines, which is free and allows you to choose from a list of feeds or link to your own, and Netvibes, which also offers links to Web-based email accounts and to social networking sites such as Facebook.

Activity 6.5 — *Reflection*

- Use a search engine to go to **www.commoncraft.com** where you will find various video clips in plain English. View any (or all) of the clips that explain the principles of Web 2.0, such as social networking, blogs, wikis, and podcasts.
- Reflect on what you have seen. Of those video clips you have viewed, which technologies do you think you would find useful?
- Go to Netvibes (**www.netvibes.com**) and scroll down the page to the 'Take a tour' link. Investigate some of the links there.
- What aspects do you think you might find useful?

Some ideas about this activity are provided at the end of the chapter.

All of these social networking skills are transferable to clinical practice, enabling you to keep in touch with fellow practitioners, building up a network of contacts and sharing experience and ideas. This will help you in your future career by making you less insular and giving you the ability to expand your horizons and learn from others, keeping up to date with information and practice.

Mobile technologies

In this third section, we will be looking at technologies that you can use when nursing in the community or on practice learning experience. The use of mobile technologies in the healthcare professions is rapidly increasing (Zurmehly, 2010). The term 'mobile technologies' encompasses the use of devices such as mobile phones, laptops, computer tablets, smart phones and Personal Digital Assistants (PDAs). Such devices are relatively small, portable and can provide easy, remote access to information.

Mobile-learning (m-learning) is learning in which mobile technologies play a central role and allow users to work away from stand-alone computers or a campus network by accessing information wirelessly. This is particularly useful to students on clinical learning opportunity and in clinical practice when out in the community.

A study at Northumbria University explored the potential for mobile technologies in supporting learning for health students. It was found that students generally use such technologies to access the internet, course materials, journals, databases, and email off-campus. Students reported that mobile technologies provide current information and improve their ability to study remotely, particularly when on practice learning opportunity. They also commented that mobile technologies facilitate increased contact with fellow students, lecturers and clinical supervisors, which reduces feelings of isolation and creates a supportive virtual environment (Walton et al., 2005).

Mobile technologies are not only used in research and education, but also in health promotion and patient care. Wider clinical applications include the ability to quickly access and update patient records, access prescription information and find current information on symptoms and treatments. Mobile phones are increasingly used to promote better nurse–patient communication, enabling the monitoring of treatment, collection of data and communication of messages for health intervention, such as the provision of support for patients attempting to give up smoking or lose weight.

Increasingly, mobile technologies are used in telemedicine, which involves using audio-visual media for consultations where the health professional and client are separated by distance. Telemedicine is used for consultations and health monitoring, and on occasion, remote medical procedures or examinations. The term telemedicine has widened to include telenursing, which could be where a nurse uses a link to a patient's television or computer in their home to provide advice and support or to monitor medication.

Not only are mobile technologies effective in providing up-to-date information but they can be cost-effective and are available at the point of care, even in remote areas. This is particularly important when working out in the community where you do not have immediate access to information via a computer or textbook. Being able to reach for a hand-held device to check diagnostic tools or patient information can make the difference between the right and wrong decision. Being able to make an informed decision is key to providing quality care for patients.

Podcasts

Podcasts are audio files that can be downloaded to mobile devices such as MP3 players, and can therefore be used anywhere. As well as being used for entertainment purposes, there are also educational applications with lecturers often recording their lectures for those who are unable to attend the session in person, audio recording of textbooks for access at any time, and libraries of downloadable sound files to aid learning, such as heart and respiratory sounds (Boulos, 2006).

Vodcasts

Videocasts, or vodcasts, work in a similar way to podcasts but are video files that can be accessed through mobile devices as well as a stand-alone PC. Although podcasts are very useful, vodcasts are perhaps a more powerful learning tool as they contain moving images which improve the learning experience.

Both podcasts and vodcasts are useful as they can be played as often as you like, repeating information to ensure retention. They also meet the needs of both auditory and visual learners and can be more interesting than reading a textbook, and therefore encourage motivation and enhance learning effectiveness.

Case study

Sean is a registered nurse working in the community and needs real-time access to information to check symptoms, diagnoses and treatment. Waiting until he gets home to use his PC isn't appropriate as it wastes time and can be detrimental to his patients. Sean remembers that he learnt about mobile technologies during his course and so buys a smart phone so that he can access the Internet while on the move. He is also able to access his email so that he can contact colleagues to double-check information and can check patient records for previous medical history. Sean manages to complete his calls for the day and feels he is on top of his workload.

Patient records

One of the biggest changes in nursing is the introduction of electronic patient records. The intention of the NHS Care Record System is to replace all paper-based medical records with a single electronic one that is updated regularly and is accessible to authorised persons and patients. Some of the advantages of electronic records include:

- currency – records can be updated immediately by health professionals, therefore providing up-to-date information;
- accuracy – entries are typed in, therefore reducing the chance of misreading information;
- availability – notes are available at any time to any member of a patient's healthcare team, even if in different locations.

Electronic records also introduce new models of care as they allow the use of care pathways and clinical networks. This isn't possible using paper records because they are often widely dispersed, sometimes not populated with the most up-to-date information, or are on occasion inaccurate due to misinterpretation of handwriting (RCN, 2006). In order to make electronic records current, accurate and accessible, they need to be updated using technologies. Certainly, some ICT skills are essential, and if out in the community, the use of mobile devices may be necessary. Records are only as useful as the information that is supplied by the healthcare professional, therefore timely and accurate input is vital and this is dependent upon your ability to make effective use of ICT. Working in the community can make you feel isolated. Mobile technologies enable you to reach out and access information remotely, keeping in contact both with colleagues and patients.

The future

In the future, the nursing workforce will continue to change, and flexibility and adaptability will be important. There will also be an increase in specialist and advanced roles. As a nurse you will therefore need to be responsive to patient needs, follow patient pathways and work across teams. You will also need to develop critical thinking skills and update your knowledge regularly (Longley, 2007). *Nursing is a unique discipline requiring complex critical thinking skills and decision making that can ultimately impact clinical competency* (Vogt, 2010, p39). Since so much information and knowledge is now available online, ICT competence allows you to access diagnostic information, interpret data, discover new therapies and techniques, document patient care and, importantly, to use current research to inform your practice and therefore support clinical decisions with sound evidence. Using those technological tools to become part of a community of practice can help in your knowledge acquisition and provide you with an important support network where you can exchange ideas. Acquiring ICT skills and learning to work with the technology is therefore a vital part of your continual professional development and will support your lifelong learning goals.

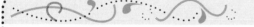

Chapter summary

This chapter has outlined information on:

- ICT skills, including Microsoft Office applications and certification alternatives;
- Web 2.0 tools, including social networking, blogs, wikis, media sharing and RSS feeds;
- mobile technologies such as mobile phones, PDAs, podcasts and vodcasts;
- nursing practice, including why ICT skills and the use of emerging technologies is important both during your studies and in nursing practice.

Activities: Brief outline answers

Activity 6.2 (page 115)

Both images were created using Excel and are well presented. Choosing between the two is a matter of your own personal preference. However, Image 2 represents the data visually as well as in a table of data. This makes the information easier to understand and more visually appealing. When presenting information, you should think about your audience. For example, if you are creating something for members of the public to see rather than medical experts, it is important to think about whether the information as you have presented it will make sense to them. Are there better ways you can explain or display things?

Activity 6.3 (page 122)

Depending on where your interests lie, there are hundreds of blogs to choose from. Some will be more useful than others and you will need to look further before deciding whether you will become a regular visitor or contributor.

The RCN blog is essentially about an initiative that takes the RCN and its resources around the UK. The first thing you may have noticed is that the latest entry was months ago. Blogs can be useful, but currency is important. Subject coverage is also an important consideration and this site seems to have very limited appeal with very little content of any real use.

Thinking about your own practice or previous experience during placement will help you to answer the question regarding the usefulness of blogs to nurses. They are only useful if they are current and if the contributor/s have something accurate and/or useful to say. Blogs are good places to share information and ideas, therefore any comments are worth reading and you can contribute your own.

Problems arise when the site isn't regularly updated and if the information is inaccurate. Do not rely on blogs alone as they may mislead or simply be someone's opinion and therefore should not be trusted. Double-check information in order to assess accuracy.

Activity 6.4 (page 123)

When consulting the ganfyd and Medpedia sites, the amount of information you find depends on the topic for which you have searched. Certainly, in terms of diabetes, the amount of content is roughly the same, therefore which you prefer is down to personal taste. Considerations to make could be: Is the site easy to search? Does the site contains images or video/audio clips that help you understand a concept more clearly? Does the site contain internal and/or external links to further information or resources? What do you think of the look and feel of the site? Again, there is no right or wrong answer – it's your own personal choice.

Activity 6.5 (page 124)

There are various video clips for you to watch and this is a useful site for clear information on technologies. The technologies you would find most useful depend on your current knowledge and perhaps your lifestyle. For example, if you have a family and little free time, playing a podcast on your MP3 player might be preferable to sitting down to read a book or journal article.

Netvibes is another site you might consider returning to in the future. Again, your choice of useful aspects is subjective, but might include social networking, widgets, media widgets, or Netvibes on your mobile.

Learning how to use technologies will encourage you to investigate further and reflect on how you might utilise that technology to acquire knowledge and to improve your practice.

Further reading

Blake, H (2008) Innovation in practice: mobile phone technology in patient care. *British Journal of Community Nursing*, 13(4): 160–5.

This article describes how mobile phones encourage better nurse–patient communication and are increasingly used in the healthcare sector.

Phillippi, JC and Buxton, M (2010) Web 2.0: easy tools for busy clinicians. *Journal of Midwifery and Women's Health*, 55(5): 472–6.

Phillippi and Buxton describe many of the Web 2.0 tools and outline how they can be used to provide evidence-based care.

Shaffer, SC, Lackey, SP and Bolling, GW (May/June 2006) Blogging as a venue for nurse faculty development. *Nursing Education Perspectives*, 126–9.

Shaffer et al. give details on how to set up a blog to meet your professional development needs, using the example of an online study group.

Skiba, DJ (2008) Nursing education 2.0: social networking for professionals. *Nursing Education Perspectives*, 29(6): 370–1.

This article introduces you to social networking for use by professionals and describes the advantages of using such tools in clinical practice.

Vogt, M et al. (2010) The impact of podcasting on the learning and satisfaction of undergraduate nursing students. *Nurse Education in Practice*, 10: 38–42.

Vogt describes in detail how podcasts can be used in nursing. The article is based on nursing education research but can be applied to a practice situation.

Walton, G, Childs, S and Blenkinsopp, E (2005) Using mobile technologies to give health students access to learning resources in the UK community setting. *Health Information and Libraries Journal*, 22 (Suppl. 2): 51–65.

Walton's article describes a project that investigated the barriers nursing students faced in using mobile technologies, and how to overcome them.

Useful websites

www.commoncraft.com

A range of video clips on Web 2.0 tools.

www.connectingforhealth.nhs.uk

This site provides information regarding the Essential IT Skills Qualification.

www.ECDL.com

The ECDL Foundation website gives information regarding ICT skills certification.

www.ehealthnurses.org.uk

This site offers information regarding IT in the NHS.

www.nmc-uk.org/Nurses-and-midwives/Advice-by-topic/A/Advice/Social-networking-sites/

The Nursing and Midwifery Council website also provides guidance on social networking.

www.wikipedia.org

This is one of the original wiki websites with a wide range of useful information, but use with caution.

Chapter 7
Information literacy: making the library work for you

Caroline Plaice and Nicola Davis

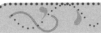 **NMC Standards for Pre-registration Nursing Education**

This chapter will address the following competencies:

Domain 1: Professional values

7. All nurses must be responsible and accountable for keeping their knowledge and skills up to date through continuing professional development. They must aim to improve their performance and enhance the safety and quality of care through evaluation, supervision and appraisal.
9. All nurses must appreciate the value of evidence in practice, be able to understand and appraise research, apply relevant theory and research findings to their work, and identify areas for further investigation.

Domain 2: Communication and interpersonal skills

8. All nurses must respect individual rights to confidentiality and keep information secure and confidential in accordance with the law and relevant ethical and regulatory frameworks, taking account of local protocols. They must also actively share personal information with others when the interests of safety and protection override the need for confidentiality.

Domain 3: Nursing practice and decision-making

1. All nurses must use up-to-date knowledge and evidence to assess, plan, deliver and evaluate care, communicate findings, influence change and promote health and best practice. They must make person-centred, evidence-based judgments and decisions, in partnership with others involved in the care process, to ensure high quality care. They must be able to recognise when the complexity of clinical decisions requires specialist knowledge and expertise, and consult or refer accordingly.
5. All nurses must understand public health principles, priorities and practice in order to recognise and respond to the major causes and social determinants of health, illness and health inequalities. They must use a range of information and data to assess the needs of people, groups, communities and populations, and work to improve health, wellbeing and experiences of healthcare; secure equal access to health screening, health promotion and healthcare; and promote social inclusion.

continued opposite . . .

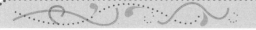

NMC Essential Skills Clusters

This chapter will address the following ESCs:

Cluster: Care, compassion and communication

7. People can trust the newly registered graduate nurse to protect and keep as confidential all information relating to them.

Cluster: Organisational aspects of care

9. People can trust the newly registered graduate nurse to treat them as partners and work with them to make a holistic and systematic assessment of their needs; to develop a personalised plan that is based on mutual understanding and respect for their individual situation promoting health and well-being, minimising risk of harm and promoting their safety at all times.

By entry to the register:

14. Applies research-based evidence to practice.

Chapter aims

By the end of this chapter you should be able to:

- understand the term 'information literacy' and its relevance to NMC competencies as a lifelong skill;
- understand the importance of a library in developing your information literacy skills;
- recognise the complementary features of physical and virtual libraries;
- understand the principles of constructing an effective literature search;
- appreciate the types of help that are available to you in using library resources both when you are in university and on practice experience.

NOTE: In this chapter we will make use of an interactive internet-based information literacy package produced by library staff at the University of the West of England, Bristol, as an exemplar of the virtual resources libraries can provide.

Introduction

When Patrice arrived at university to start her nursing degree, she thought her tutors would give her all the information she needed to pass her exams. It came as a shock to hear that most of the skills she needed she would learn in practice experience, and the majority of information she needed would come from her own research carried out using the resources available through the Health and Social Care Library on campus. One of the essential skills for any nurse to develop within their studies is the ability to find and use evidence effectively to inform healthcare decision-making. The NMC (2008) is clear that it is extremely important for all concerned that the best available evidence informs clinical practice. Knowing how to locate, evaluate and synthesise evidence are lifelong skills. Developing those skills starts at the beginning of your course when you have a great opportunity to engage in a dialogue with your library service. Building your confidence and competence in using the library and its resources now, means that when you need information when you are out in practice, you will be able to search quickly and effectively for evidence on which to make decisions.

Developing your information literacy (IL) skills

Libraries provide resources and support to enable you to start your information literacy journey.

Information literacy [involves] knowing when and why you need information, where to find it, and how to evaluate, use and communicate it in an ethical manner
(CILIP, 2010).

Its importance was highlighted by US President Barack Obama when he stated that:

we dedicate ourselves to increasing information literacy awareness so that all citizens understand its vital importance. An informed and educated citizenry is essential to the functioning of our modern democratic society . . .
(quoted in Godwin, 2009).

Further, UNESCO declared that IL:

is a basic human right in the digital world as it empowers individuals in all walks of life to seek, evaluate, use and create information effectively to achieve their personal, social, occupational and educational goals
(Godwin, 2009).

It is helpful to look a little more at what actually constitutes IL. The Society of College, National and University Libraries (SCONUL) (2007) identifies 'seven pillars of information literacy' consisting of the following steps.

1. Recognise an information need.
2. Distinguish ways of addressing the gap.
3. Construct strategies for locating.
4. Locate and access.
5. Compare and evaluate.
6. Organise, apply and communicate.
7. Synthesise and communicate.

In this chapter, within the context of your first year of nursing studies, we will concentrate on the third and fourth pillars of information literacy. These skills are among the most important to develop at the beginning of your studies. But first, let us consider the basics – how can you use the library?

Activity 7.1	*Evidence-based practice and research*

It is invaluable to familiarise yourself with the way your library works. Spend a few minutes finding answers to these questions. They can also be found on the iSkillZone website (see Useful websites at the end of the chapter) if you want to find out more.

- What do you need to provide in order to join your library?
- What time is the library open, both in term time and during vacation? (There are normally longer opening hours in term time.)
- How are the shelves organised? This might be by Dewey Decimal Classification where the nursing titles start at 610.73, or by another method.
- If you find a resource on the catalogue that is already on loan, how do you go about reserving it?

As this is based on your own research, there is no outline answer provided.

How did you get on? You might want to discuss your results with your peers or tutor. Find out more about how the library can support you on your journey by reading on.

Physical and virtual libraries

Libraries are increasingly providing resources and support electronically. Many university libraries provide thousands of resources in this way, but libraries provide much more than this. Walk into your library and you will find sources of help and comfortable workspaces as well as resources. It is really worth the effort of going into the library at the start of your course to check this out.

As part of your journey, you can discover something about yourself: what kind of learner you are and what kind of space you prefer to work in – whether in silence or through group study. Most libraries or learning centres provide areas for group discussion (including the viewing of, for example, DVDs), or more discreet spaces for quiet study and silent work. Make the effort to familiarise yourself with the physical library space and you may well be rewarded by finding out which suits you best, and when it is available. Many libraries have invested thoughtfully in creating pleasant and attractive spaces in which you can think and work in comfort and relative peace. Make the most of these spaces – it may well be that distractions from learning can be contained better when you work in the library, especially as your telephone will not be ringing!

Other features to look out for in the physical library include current journals – why not pull up a chair or log on to a key title and have a browse through the current hot topics? Have a look around the shelves in the area where resources on your subject are located and get a feel for the types of literature that are available. Become a good 'library detective' and you may stumble across some really useful resources through serendipity. Many libraries provide informative displays showcasing their new resources in a particular subject area. Some have themed displays to tie in with, for example, NHS 'weeks' on topics such as depression, HIV/AIDS awareness or smoking cessation. These can provide you with inspiration on a topic and help you focus your thinking on a piece of learning. You may be able to find information to help a patient you are caring for in your practice experience.

You might be surprised at the number of hours the library is available to you every day, even when library staff are not there. In many libraries you will be able to use self-service facilities. By becoming familiar with the physical library, you will also have the opportunity to get to meet library staff, who are there to help and advise you. Find out if there is a particular librarian who supports your course as they may have specialist interests. You may get to meet the librarians at an induction at the beginning of your learning journey. Your library may have help points where you can ask a question, or make an appointment for more extensive help with a member of staff Some libraries provide drop-in sessions, lunchtime workshops, even Saturday surgeries where you can get help from a member of library staff on issues such as database searching or reference management. In addition, there may be online sources of help – for example, an 'Ask a Librarian' service on the library web pages where you can post a question and a member of library staff will respond to you within a specified time. Finding out this information early on in your course is invaluable; you can then feel confident to use the library and its staff in the most effective manner.

Scenario

Your colleague Abdul has unfortunately missed his library tour because his travel arrangements from Uganda were disrupted and he couldn't get to the course induction until day 4. The library talk, which included an orientation quiz and treasure hunt, had been on day 3. You found the induction really helpful and inspiring, and want to help Abdul benefit as well. How could Abdul catch up on this valuable experience?

There are a number of ways in which Abdul could have found out about the library. Many libraries have virtual tours of their spaces so you can orientate yourself and find out more about the opening hours and services available. Have a look at **www.uwe.ac.uk/library** for an example. In Abdul's case, there was also a podcast available from the library website introducing him to the Liaison Librarian for his programme as well as a link to a blog to find out more about current events and news in the library. In addition, he received an email invitation to follow the library on Twitter, and this provided information about some additional sessions for the orientation quiz and treasure hunt too. These had been organised when the faculty librarian realised that ten other people on Abdul's course had had similar travel problems.

Sources of support on your practice learning opportunities

It can be difficult to access your university library when you are out on practice. There are a number of ways, however, in which you can get help. First, find out what support the library provides for students on placement. This might include photocopying articles, posting out books and holding items on reserve for you to collect. Note that there may be an administration charge for some of these services. Some libraries provide the services of an 'outreach' or 'placement' librarian, who will visit clinical placement areas. Don't forget e-books too – they can be invaluable when you are off site, accessible via the internet. In addition, you may find the university library provides helpful advice on useful websites.

> ## Case study
>
> *Heather needed information on infection control to help her prepare for a seminar on MRSA. The librarian showed her how to use the new search facility on the catalogue to search the resources held physically in the library and those held electronically in journals to which the library subscribes. It did not take long to locate several up-to-date resources that helped in her research. Heather found recent statistics on MRSA infection and the evidence for best practice in controlling its spread. She was able to disseminate this important information to her fellow students, who will know how to combat this infection when in practice.*

Apart from these university services, your first year and early placements are the time to find out what your NHS library can provide – you will be able to join one while on placement – and this gives you access to a further wide range of resources, which will complement those provided by the university. Bearing in mind you may eventually take up a post in the NHS, it is extremely valuable to find out about the resources you can use in this setting.

Types of resources and how to locate them

You will probably have been given a list of resources your tutor would like you to read and consider. This may have included books, journal articles and other materials, and may be available in a range of formats – print, as part of a digital collection, or as an electronic book (e-book). If the resource is available as part of your course information, you may find it is posted on a **virtual learning environment**. Otherwise, your best bet is to use the library catalogue to locate it.

Books

The library catalogue provides you with details of all the books your library has. Generally, catalogues are available via the internet, so you can search from any web-enabled computer to find a catalogue such as the one at **www.uwe.ac.uk/library/catalogue**. Type in the link and take a look, if you can. Figure 7.1 overleaf shows what a page from the catalogue looks like.

Catalogues let you search in a number of ways, usually by author, title or key word. You do not need to know all a book's details in order to find it. There may also be a link for searching for specific media, such as e-books and anatomical models, as well as any special collections – for example, a 'user participation collection'. Once you have located the book you are interested in there will be a link for further information and this will show you which library the title is held in and whether any copies are available. You may be able to reserve a copy if the one you want is on loan. Increasingly, the trend is also for the further details section to include the contents page of the book and sometimes a commercial review of the book. If the title is available electronically,

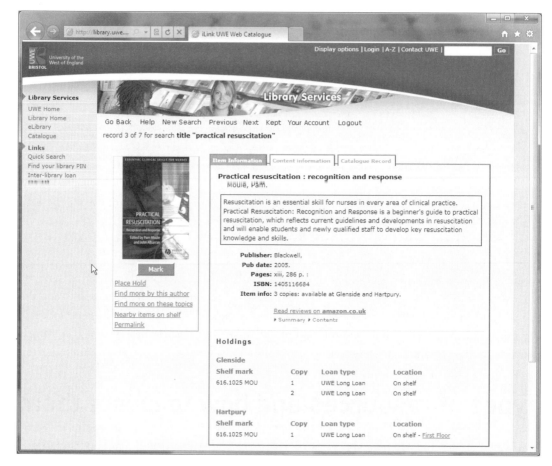

Figure 7.1: A page from a library catalogue

there will be a message along the lines of 'connect to resource', which will link you straight to the item. You will probably need to sign in at this stage using the user name and password assigned to you at the beginning of your course.

Electronic books

This is an increasingly popular medium. An electronic book (e-book) is either a digitised copy of a book available in print or a book only available in electronic form, sometimes known as 'born digital'. You read it via a computer screen or an e-book reader. The advantage of using an e-book is that it is available whenever and wherever you need it via your library website. This is particularly useful when you cannot get into the library or when you are on practice experience. Just like a print book, copyright legislation guidelines mean that you can only print a percentage, and some e-book platforms also limit the amount of time you can store the book on your PC or laptop (normally a maximum of 24 hours).

Not all books are available electronically, but increasingly libraries are buying e-books as part of their digital strategy (this book is available as an e-book). If you are using the library catalogue, you will find e-books along with other resources, but if you are browsing the shelves, it might not be apparent that there is an e-resource available. This is why it is so important to make effective use of the catalogue and, of course, you can always ask a member of library staff to clarify how to do this if you are not sure.

Journals

Journals are also known as serials or periodicals (because they are published periodically). They are published by academic institutions, organisations and commercial publishers, either weekly, monthly, bi-monthly, quarterly or annually. Journals are a very important source of information because, unlike books, they provide a regular source of up-to-date information. In addition, the information is not generally held elsewhere; it may contain the opinions of experts in their specific field as well as research findings. Importantly, journals usually contain a list of references at the end, which direct you to further information. Increasingly, the journals that libraries buy are available as 'electronic journals' as well or exclusively, which means they are accessible over the internet. Most libraries subscribe to an increasing array of electronic journal titles, so check the catalogue to see what is available. There will probably be an 'A–Z of electronic titles' you can browse, or go to a specific title which has been recommended to you. Print journals are generally restricted to library use only and cannot be borrowed.

Journals generally fall into two types: academic and professional. Academic journals, such as the *British Medical Journal*, are often quite specialised and written by academics or subject specialists. These journals will usually be peer-reviewed, which means that the quality of an article has been rigorously assessed by other specialists in the field before it appears in print. Academic journals normally follow a pattern. They provide an abstract, introduction, review of literature, findings, conclusion and list of references. Professional journals, such as *Nursing Times*, are generally more practice-orientated. They may include updates and general information for practitioners as well as discussions about policy areas, short research reports and job advertisements for professionals in that field.

Activity 7.2   *Evidence-based practice and research*

This activity focuses on understanding more about journals. You will need to consult the journals collection in your library.

- Find three peer-reviewed nursing journals and make a note of the titles. Information on whether a journal is peer reviewed usually appears at the beginning of the journal.
- Note down the title of three professional journals to which your library subscribes.
- Are these titles held in print, electronic form or both?
- Find the abstract of two articles that interest you in the peer-reviewed journals.
- Print out the articles. They may be useful in the future.

Alternatively, try the short interactive quiz on journals available from the iSkillZone website. Go to **http://iskillzone.uwe.ac.uk/** and click on 'finding journal articles'.

As this is based on your own research, there is no outline answer provided.

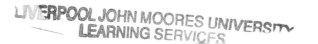

We will cover how to find journal articles on a particular topic later in this chapter (see pages 140–1).

Other resources

Bear in mind that there may be resources available to you other than books and journals. DVDs are very popular and some health and social care libraries have large collections, including fiction and drama-based films, which can be borrowed for both individual and group viewing. Some libraries have staff dedicated to identifying and recording healthcare-related television broadcasts, such as documentaries and speeches. Some health libraries also have anatomical models (see Figure 7.2), which are a useful, engaging adjunct to other learning materials and an excellent way of enhancing group presentations (you may be able to borrow them for a short period of time). The next activity aims to help you reflect on the wide variety of resources to augment your learning that are available in the library.

Activity 7.3   *Evidence-based practice and research*

Find out whether your library makes off-air recordings of health-related television programmes and how you can request that a specific programme of interest is recorded. Make a note of the programmes already in the library that you would like to watch.

As this is based on your own research, there is no outline answer provided.

There is a growing trend to 'stream' programmes so they can be viewed over the internet at a later date and your library may have invested in this new technology to make multimedia resources available to you in this way.

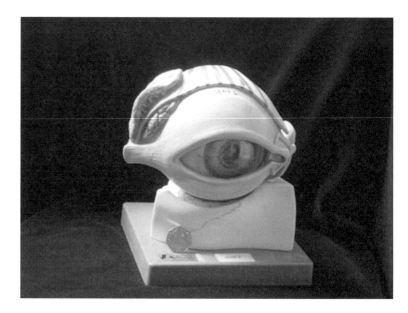

Figure 7.2: Anatomical model of an eye

Searching for information on specific subjects

As an information literate person you must be able to recognise when there is a gap in your knowledge and therefore when information is needed. Beyond that it is also critically important to have the ability to find, critique and consider whether or how to use the required information effectively. As part of this process you need to define the purpose and scope of your project, as well as considering what or who the information is for. You might consider what type of document your work will become, what level of detail is needed and indeed, who will read your work. All of these considerations could influence how much information will be needed.

Planning a literature search

If you have a topic to search, but don't have any specific sources in mind, a journal search is one of the best first places to start. But what is the best way to go about it? One of the key elements of successful assignment writing is having sufficient time to plan, refine and carry out your literature search effectively. The box below contains a suggested project plan to facilitate your search.

Plan for literature search

1. If you have been given a broad topic on which to search, decide on the initial topic by browsing books and journals on the library catalogue. Also look at the relevant sections in the library. The time you have invested in getting to know your library layout, familiarising yourself with the catalogue as well as finding out the sources of support available to you will be invaluable here.
2. Look at relevant websites. The NHS Evidence portal (www.evidence.nhs.uk) is invaluable here.
3. Once you have a firmer idea of the topic, create a mind map of key words. An example of a mind map is shown in Figure 7.3 on page 142.
4. Carry out an initial search using the library's **federated search** facility.
5. Refine your keywords. ·
6. If you are carrying out an extended piece of writing, set up an **electronic alert** (see page 148) so you can be informed when new articles in your area of interest are published.
7. Refine your search using individual or **native databases** and make use of advanced searching techniques.
8. Save your references into a **bibliographic management software** package for later use.
9. Request any journal articles that are relevant but not held in the library.
10. Write the assignment and add the reference list.

We will describe and discuss the stages of this plan in more detail below, but first we will reflect a little more about the resources you will be using to search for information on a topic.

Databases

The most efficient current way to search for journal articles is via databases. A database is like a filing cabinet indexing thousands of journals, which means that in essence someone else has done some of the hard work for you. But where do you start? There are at least three core databases with which you need to become familiar; they should all be included as a foundation for all your searches.

CINAHL, the Cumulative Index to Nursing and Allied Health Literature, is a key resource for nursing, midwifery and the allied health professions. It is produced in the USA and indexes over 2,800 journals from around the world. So this is a very large database with an international focus.

BNI, British Nursing Index is another important resource for nursing and midwifery. It indexes over 200 major UK journals, and subjects covered include both general and specialist nursing areas.

MEDLINE is the largest database in the health sciences. It contains over 11 million references from almost 5,000 international journals, and subjects covered include medicine, dentistry, veterinary medicine and medical psychology.

Authors may sometimes write in journals indexed in databases outside of these core databases. So you may need to think laterally, depending on your topic, and search databases with more of a European medical emphasis, such as Embase, or maybe those with a more psychological perspective such as PsycInfo. Social Care Online, which is an important source of social care information (**www.scie-socialcareonline.org.uk/**) and contains additional information as well as a database of articles. The links to policy documents and e-learning resources are particularly useful.

You need to consider how you can make the best and most efficient use of these databases, so that they work hard for you and save you valuable time. Remember that all these licensed resources will require you to 'authenticate' yourself, or log in using a specific user name and password. Ask in the library if you are not sure whether you have this. Do not wait until you have a pressing deadline for an essay when you might not be able to find out your personal log-in details in time.

Specialist resources

The databases referred to above cover a range of information sources on a wide variety of topics. There are other source-specific resources that can be very useful to explore. They include the resources in the Cochrane Library, a collection of six databases that contain different types of high-quality, independent evidence and constitute a key source of information on the effectiveness of healthcare interventions. Among them is a storehouse of systematic reviews, sometimes referred to as 'platinum standard evidence' and comprised of secondary sources. You can find out more about the nature and components of secondary sources in Chapter 8.

Other examples of source-specific resources are those that concentrate on other types of secondary source such as clinical guidelines. These make use of wide consultancy and the systematic reviews produced, for example, by Cochrane, to develop guidance for practice. One example is the work of the Scottish Intercollegiate Guidelines Network (SIGN) found at **www.sign.ac.uk/index.html**.

You might also choose to look at NHS Evidence, the NHS portal of information that can be found at **www.evidence.nhs.uk**. This provides access to a wide range of resources and government policy. One of the most useful areas within this information resource is the Specialist Collections, which pull together resources on a variety of healthcare conditions, topics and considerations of health populations. Many of the resources within NHS Evidence are freely available, although some are restricted to those with NHS authentication.

In Chapter 9 a case study (page 187) asks you to reflect on a staff nurse's experience of a clinical incident concerning a man who was recovering from a myocardial infarction who goes into cardiac arrest. One of the issues raised was the Senior Nurse's disregard for correct manual handling procedures. Read through the case study and use NHS Evidence to find what evidence is available to support staff in raising concerns about adherence to manual handling policy.

An outline answer is provided at the end of the chapter

Choosing your search terms and creating a mind map

When you want to find the best sources of evidence to support your studies and practice, you need to engage thoughtfully and thoroughly in searching within the databases available to you. One of the first considerations is how you think your specific topic might be referred to. Take pressure sores as an example. These wounds might also be referred to as pressure ulcers, bed sores, or decubitus ulcers. Knowing that topics may be referred to in a variety of ways helps us to think about how many search terms and phrases might be needed to carry out a thorough literature review. Consider the topic of older people and pressure sores. The diagram below gives an example of how you might plan to capture all of the synonyms or alternate words for this topic. Don't forget that language can change over time; we might be more comfortable using the phrase 'older person' but in the past 'geriatrics' would have been used more widely, so include that in your mind map. The mind map in Figure 7.3 was generated by the Inspiration package (see Useful websites).

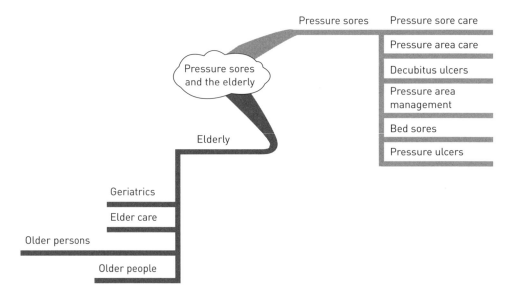

Figure 7.3: A mind map on pressure sores and the elderly

Activity 7.5   *Evidence-based practice and research*

Abdul has been asked to write an assignment on the issues surrounding the presence of a patient's relatives at cardio-pulmonary resuscitation. Create a mind map to show the keywords and phrases that you might want to use.

A sample answer is provided at the end of the chapter.

Creating the 'funnel-shaped search'

You might not have heard of a literature search being described in terms of a shape before. What we mean in this context is that you can make use of the strategies available to you within the databases in order to locate as many potential sources as possible in your initial searches. In doing so, you may stand every chance of being able to 'catch' the sources of most relevance to your topic. If we were to use an analogy here we might compare this process to fishing. You might want to catch salmon; you will need to cast the net wide to catch them and initially they may be mixed with other types of fish that you simply don't want. So you need to be able to make effective use of the databases so that the extraneous literature is 'filtered' out as soon as possible.

Federated searching

At this initial stage, try searching across several databases at once. This is known as 'federated searching' and allows you to simultaneously search the literature across BNI, CINAHL and MEDLINE, among many other databases. It does not allow particularly sophisticated searching, or support advanced searching techniques, but it is an important starting point and helps to identify which databases will be of most use later on. This is because a federated search will show you how many hits each of the databases has found in total.

A federated search may also help you refine your mind map by pointing to keywords that had not initially been part of your map. Look at the full view of the records you've found using the federated search engine. Under 'key words' or 'subject headings' you'll be able to see the words or phrases the indexers considered to be the most important elements of the article and which have been assigned as 'tags' to the piece of writing to help in retrieving it.

Google Scholar

It would be useful at this stage to discuss the facility provided by Google Scholar. You might be thinking, 'Why can't I just use that to do all my searching?' Well, there is certainly a place for this search engine and colleagues have sometimes described it as 'a guilty pleasure', but it has some disadvantages too. Google Scholar is not comprehensive and you may not find the literature you need for your topic, but you won't be sure that is the case because you will only know what you have found, not what you missed.

In addition, Google Scholar doesn't always distinguish between high quality academic writing and other types of unsubstantiated literature, which might be inappropriate or even dangerous

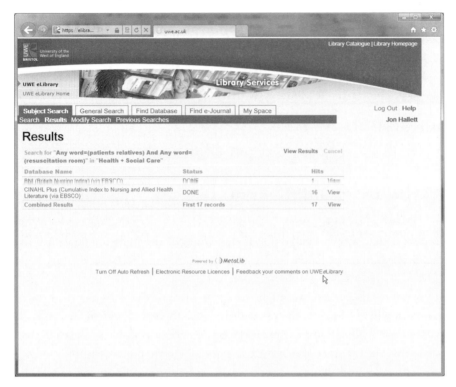

Figure 7.4: Search results from each individual database

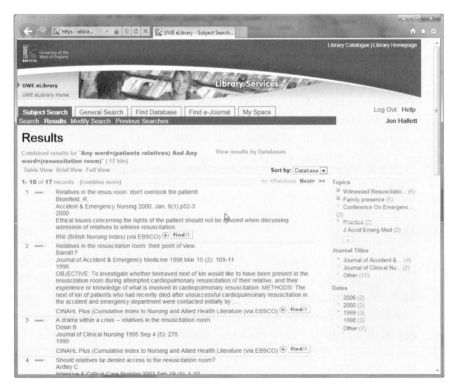

Figure 7.5: A federated search of e-library using 'patients' and 'relatives'

for you to use. Neither will it tell you how to distinguish between good and bad evidence. Finally, the articles you find via this engine may be difficult to access because the site in question does not recognise you as a bona fide user. In summary, use this facility only in moderation. Try not to use it as the only form of support for any of your literature searching because you might come unstuck and not find what you need.

Refining your search

Having carried out an initial search, you now need to filter through your results.

Porter (2008) discusses the 'funnel-shaped search' to remind us that the numbers of hits or articles located might start large but we cannot manage the process effectively if the numbers stay large. After casting the net wide to catch all potential 'treasure', you need to make use of advanced search techniques and filtering in order to get the 'hit' numbers under control. Depending on which subject you need to explore, the numbers of potential papers might be very high, far too high to screen the abstracts of every paper.

Basic searching can be useful in 'testing out' your search terms. You could view this as a scoping exercise to identify the breadth and range of potential papers useful to your study. Even within simple searching you may be able to hone down your search to year of publication, journal title and author. Your tutor will almost certainly ask you to limit your search to up-to-date information, so restricting to articles published within the last five years is an example of limiting your search.

Straightforward combinations of search terms or search phrases can be used even with simple searches. This simple process can quickly initiate some specificity within the search, which might be very helpful in keeping the number of hits within manageable limits right from the very start. So with Abdul's research on patient resuscitation, he may decide to be more specific and only consider articles that look at the presence of siblings, rather than relatives in general, in the resuscitation room.

Using native databases to refine your search

Once you have carried out your initial search, it is the time to move on to individual or 'native' databases. BNI, CINAHL and MEDLINE are examples of individual databases. These allow you to employ more advanced searching techniques. As well as planning the key words, alternative words and synonyms, you can now start to refine your search. There are a number of ways you can do this. Truncation is a technique to employ in ensuring the tenacity of the 'completeness' of the initial searches, so essentially it is useful at the top of the funnel. This search technique refers to the capacity to search for all variants of a word. Typically, a symbol such as '*' or '$' is used to represent the rest of the term, inserted at the root where a word may be subject to change. Different databases prefer the asterisk or the dollar sign, so check which one is needed in each case. End truncation is where several letters at the beginning of a word are specified but the ending can vary. This may be very important where perhaps the topic foci include words subject to such change. An example of this would be a topic like how to 'communicate with patients', because if you truncate 'communicat*', you may pick up on papers that discuss communication, communicating, communicates, etc. Stemming is a term that relates to truncation. It usually refers to the ability of a search engine to find variations of a word changed by features such as plurals, singular forms, tense, etc.

End truncation	nurs*	Finds: nurse, nurses, nursing, nursed
Internal truncation/wildcard	bl*d	Finds: blood, bled, bleed

Table 7.1: Examples of truncation

A word of caution here, though: sometimes using truncation can have unwanted results – for instance, using child* would include childbirth as well as child, children, childhood, so think carefully before applying truncation. You might have to accept that you may still have to 'weed out' some extraneous hits.

Another form of refinement can be applied by using Boolean Operators. Distinct from truncation, the use of Boolean Operators can either broaden or narrow a search depending on which word is employed. Boolean Searching refers to a process wherein multiple terms are combined in a search.

and	requires that both terms be found within the search; AND will therefore narrow it
or	allows either term be found, so will **BROADEN** the search
not	means any record containing the second term will be excluded, which can be very useful in selective exclusion of certain facets, e.g. pre-operative fasting 'not' child*

Table 7.2: Examples of using Boolean Operators

An example could look like this:

1. leg ulcer* and honey
2. older person or older people or elder*
3. 1 and 2

This search strategy would therefore find articles about the treatment of leg ulcers with honey in older people.

Let's try out some of these techniques using the example of one of the assignment topics mentioned previously: family-witnessed resuscitation. You would commence with an initial search using a federated search engine available from the library. Having found some results provides you with lots of ideas about the exact topic you want to focus on – and helps you think of other terms that might be useful. You decide to focus on relatives in the resuscitation room, specifically focused on one age group, in this case with children. Your planning enables you to come up with the following strategy that you run in a native database.

Key concept: relatives	Key concept: resuscitation room	Key concept: child
relatives family sibling* parent* family member* next of kin spectator* family presen* grandparent* brother* sister*	resuscitation room witnessed resuscitation emergency room young child*	child* teenage* infant

Table 7.3: Developing your search strategy

Run the first key concept first. So, on the first line, you'd type in 'relatives', the second 'family' and so on all the way to sister* which would be search 11. Using your Boolean Operator 'or' you would then combine all of these terms by saying '1 or 2 or 3' up to search 11. This means that the database search engine will search for occurrences of any of these alternative words.

Then you can move on to the second key concept, that of the resuscitation room. Again, run each concept and then put them together using the 'or' operator. Once you have completed all the key concepts you can then use the 'and' operator to put it all together. This will mean that at least one key concept from each of your three categories will appear in your search results.

The default in the database for searching for your key concepts is usually the title, author and abstract fields of the article. You can also look at the controlled vocabulary or thesaurus facility of a database to provide you with more information on subject headings.

How not to 'dent the funnel'

Do not be seduced by the 'full text only' button. This strategy would only reveal journals that your library has paid for in full electronic form and this can vary for many reasons. Therefore, if you tick the box for full text only, you have inadvertently introduced an element of chance that you may not want to risk. You might just be excluding the paper that you really need before your search has really 'found its feet'. Similarly, you do not want to tick the box for research only. It cannot be relied upon because it might lead to papers that are someone else's interpretation of what constitutes research or just to a paper that mentions research. It is no guarantee of automatically finding a primary source.

Regarding articles located in journals to which your library does not subscribe, do remember that you can request extra papers via the library **inter-library loan system** and you may not even be charged for that if you keep the requests within reasonable limits. So if you allow enough time to complete your search early, you should have the time to make such requests.

Snowballing

Snowball literature searching can be an exciting way of advancing your understanding of the complexity of certain topics, including identifying the major theorists writing within the topic area. You might also uncover a group of experts, who refer to each other.

Activity 7.6   *Evidence-based practice and research*

- Consider how you might find the most recent articles on your topic.
- Find two of the articles cited in that paper.
- Find out how you can search forward in time – how can you find papers that have cited the papers you have found?
- Are there any key authors?

An outline answer is given at the end of the chapter.

Setting up alerts

If you are carrying out an extended essay over time, you may want to set up an electronic alert so that you can be informed every time an article is published in your defined topic area. Follow the online instructions within the database you are using to do this. You will need to register your details (name, email address etc.) so that the service can email you the relevant articles. If you find that you aren't getting the kind of articles you expected, then you may need to refine your search terms or phrases.

Exporting your references

Once you have become fluent with your search techniques, you will have found lots of references and will need to start drawing the information and ideas together. Many libraries provide access to packages that allow you to export and save the details of the references you have found and organise them into folders. Once you have carried out a search you can select the relevant articles you want to save by exporting them into the package. This is a really efficient way of organising the information you have found and will save you time when you have completed your assignment and are checking to ensure you have fully referenced the sources you have cited within your work.

Referencing and avoiding plagiarism

> *Referencing: (is) the means of telling your reader where you found the information you've used in a piece of work*
> (iSkillZone, 2008).

Correct and accurate referencing is an integral part of writing your essay and enables a reader to refer back to the sources you have used to gain more information or to check a specific point. A key element of your academic journey and information management skills set is to gain

competence and confidence with referencing. Unfortunately, there isn't one single way of referencing, but rather several different approaches. As soon as you can, identify which reference
system is currently used where you are studying. Arguably the most oft found referencing system,
which uses the author and title method, is known as the Harvard system and gives full details of
each source at the end of the article; the Vancouver system uses a numbering in the text with the
details listed at the end. It is important that you check with your tutors which one they use because
your ability to reference correctly will be one of the skills that they assess in your work.

Activity 7.7 — *Critical thinking*

Remember the journal articles you found in Activity 7.2 (page 137)? Create a reference list
using these titles in the Harvard style of referencing. To practise referencing a variety
of media types, you might like to consider referencing a website, book and DVD on your
topic too.

If you have access, work through the 'referencing' section of the iSkillZone at **http://
iskillzone.uwe.ac.uk**. This facility will explain how to reference correctly and why it is
so important within your academic work.

There are some example reference lists at the end of this chapter.

You will have discovered in Activity 7.7 that referencing is so important in terms of showing
due respect for other people's work. You are sharing your understanding of their ideas, but
their contribution to your thinking should be acknowledged. To do otherwise could justify an
accusation of taking other people's work or ideas, which is a form of plagiarism. Plagiarism is
an academic offence that can be regarded as an assessment offence if found in your work,
with disciplinary consequences. It can easily be avoided. iSkillZone contains more information
on this.

Chapter summary

Within this chapter we have sought to share with you a great enthusiasm for the library and
all that it can offer. The virtual library is flexible and accessible if you have internet access,
but you may need training as to how to make the best use of this facility. The physical
library offers you so much more than books; it may be your preferred site of learning as
well as a treasure store of diverse resources including multimedia items. There is almost
certainly going to be something in the library to meet every learner's needs. However, in
order to make the best use of your library you need to learn and refine information literacy
skills. Once you have mastered the ability to identify and respond to your own knowledge
gaps, you may well be amazed by how much the library can assist and advise you. This can
include helping you to manage your references, keep track of your sources and cite them
correctly.

Activities: Brief outline answers

Activity 7.4 (page 142)

By searching on 'manual handling procedures' you will find items such as the Resuscitation Council Guidance for safer handling during resuscitation in healthcare settings (2009), which will enable you to raise your concerns using evidence-based sources. There are also some key primary sources written on this topic available via CINAHL.

Activity 7.5 (page 143)

Your mind map might look something like this.

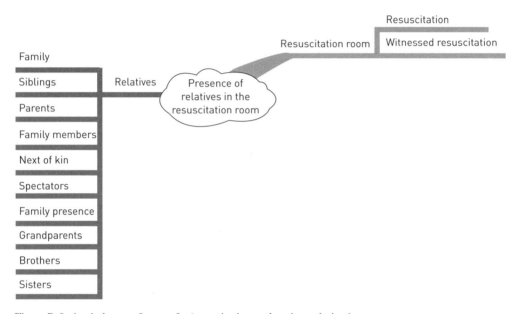

Figure 7.6: A mind map of terms for 'resuscitation and patient relatives'

Activity 7.6 (page 148)

The best place to start a search for articles is using a federated search, which allows you to search a range of databases that contain journal literature. Think about the key terms that express your concepts and to find the most recent article limit your search to the last two years of articles published. To carry out a more detailed search, go to a native database. The search you performed initially will be helpful in constructing your literature search strategy by providing ideas on the key words or phrases that articles on the topic you are interested in have been arranged.

Your library may have the article you've found either in print or electronically. If it doesn't, request it through the inter-library loan service. Once you have the article, look at the references at the end. Select a couple and make a note of the details of the reference: the author(s), title of article, title of journal and the date, volume, issue number (if there is one) and page numbers of the article. You can then go back to the library catalogue and carry out a journal search for that title. If the title is held in the library for that year, you can then find the article on the shelf, or if it is held electronically, click to connect to the electronic resource. While libraries have a vast array of resources, they don't have access to every journal you might find. You might want to look at alternative references if the one you have located is not accessible, or request a copy from another library, for which there may be a charge. One really useful resource to use is the Journal

Citation Index. This allows you to search forwards in the literature. So, you could use this database to see whether anyone has quoted the paper you originally found. This can lead you to further relevant sources of information.

Finally, be vigilant as to multiple occurrences of particular authors on a subject; the same author may come up a number of times in the article you have found, which could well indicate he or she is an expert in the field. You could go back to your federated search engine and search for this particular author to check whether they have written more on the field in which you are interested.

Activity 7.7 (page 149)

Here are some examples of Harvard referencing for different media types on the topic of 'communication, equity and diversity'. Always check with your tutor the form of referencing you are required to use.

Journal article

Piki, E (2010) Cultural diversity. *Nursing Standard* 24 (29): 1–2.

Cross, W M and Bloomer, M J (2010) Extending boundaries: clinical communication with culturally and linguistically diverse mental health clients and carers. *International Journal of Mental Health Nursing* 19 (4): 268–77.

Electronic journal article

Narayanasamy, A (2005) A review of transcultural nursing. *Nurse Education Today* 2005, 25(2): 102–11 (online) DOI:10.1016/j.nedt.2004.09.011 (accessed 23 November 2010).

Book

Moss, B (2008) *Communication Skills for Health and Social Care*. London: Sage.

Website

Department of Health (2010). *Equity and excellence: Liberating the NHS* (online). Available from: www.dh.gov.uk/en/Healthcare/LiberatingtheNHS/index.htm (accessed 24 November 2010).

DVD

Getting on: series one (2009) DVD. Directed by Peter Capaldi. London: BBC.

Further reading

Bowling, A and Ebrahim, S (eds) (2005) *Handbook of Health Research Methods: Investigation, measurement and analysis*. Berkshire: Open University Press.

This is a well written and accessible overview of research designs that healthcare students need to know about.

Gray, A and Harrison, S (2004) *Governing Medicine: Theory and practice*. Berkshire, Open University Press.

This is a particularly insightful discussion of the political and professional implications of clinical governance.

Hutchfield, K (2010) *Information Skills for Nursing Students*. Exeter: Learning Matters.

A practical and clear guide to finding, assessing, retrieving and storing information for nursing course work and practice.

Moule, P and Goodman, M (2009) *Nursing Research: An introduction*. London: Sage Publications.

A well-written and accessible overview of nursing research designs, including a glossary and user-friendly critiquing framework.

Rumsey, S (2004) *How to find Information*. Berkshire: Open University Press.

An accessible text that focuses on developing information literacy skills in some detail.

White, M (2007) *Making Search Work*. London: Facet Publishing.

An accessible text that focuses on developing information literacy skills in more detail.

Useful websites

http://iskillzone.uwe.ac.uk

The iSkillZone from the University of the West of England, Bristol, is an interactive information literacy tool that is freely available for use over the internet. This section highlights the importance of journals and how to use them effectively.

www.evidence.nhs.uk

This website is the first stop for accessing the wide range of resources available to those working in health and social care to assist in providing quality patient care.

www.inspiration.com

A visual learning tool software package that is really useful for creating mind maps.

www.sign.ac.uk

The Scottish Intercollegiate Guidelines Network is an excellent example of guidelines that have been developed to assist in clinical decision-making.

www.scie-socialcareonline.org.uk

This website gives access to the UK's most complete range of information and research on all aspects of social care and social work.

www.uwe.ac.uk/library

This is an example of a university library home page. It acts as a starting point from which to find information on what is available (including the catalogue), check opening hours, request interlibrary loans, search databases and post questions to librarians.

Chapter 8
Evidence-based practice: aspiring to achieve quality

Nicola Davis

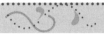

NMC Standards for Pre-registration Nursing Education

This chapter will address the following competencies:

Domain 1: Professional values

9. All nurses must appreciate the value of evidence in practice, be able to understand and appraise research, apply relevant theory and research findings to their work, and identify areas for further investigation.

Domain 3: Nursing practice and decision-making

1. All nurses must use up-to-date knowledge and evidence to assess, plan, deliver and evaluate care, communicate findings, influence change and promote health and best practice. They must make person-centred, evidence-based judgments and decisions, in partnership with others involved in the care process, to ensure high quality care. They must be able to recognise when the complexity of clinical decisions requires specialist knowledge and expertise, and consult or refer accordingly.

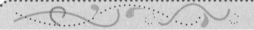

NMC Essential Skills Clusters

This chapter will address the following ESCs:

Cluster: Organisational aspects of care

9. People can trust the newly registered graduate nurse to treat them as partners and work with them to make a holistic and systematic assessment of their needs; to develop a personalised plan that is based on mutual understanding and respect for their individual situation promoting health and well-being, minimising risk of harm and promoting their safety at all times.

By entry to the register:

14. Applies research-based evidence to practice.

16. People can trust the newly registered graduate nurse to safely lead, co-ordinate and manage care.

continued overleaf . . .

continued . . .

> *By entry to the register:*
>   3. Bases decisions on evidence and uses experience to guide decision-making.

Chapter aims

By the end of this chapter, you should be able to:

*   understand where evidence can be found, and how to construct an effective literature search to find evidence;
*   identify types of sources of evidence and know how to recognise them;
*   know the fundamental questions to include in critiques of primary, secondary and tertiary sources, moving towards critical appraisal;
*   discuss why evidence-based practice matters in terms of practising in line with NMC regulation and clinical governance;
*   understand the concept of advocacy: acting in the client's best interests and dealing with challenges to evidence-based practice.

Introduction

Case study

Staff Nurse Baker is a firm believer that all patients should be washed, dressed and sitting in the chairs next to their beds by 10 a.m. every morning. That is how it was done when she did her training. She is called in to speak to the Ward Manager one afternoon because a client's family has made a complaint against her. Apparently, the client has developed a sore sacrum and the family are complaining that this is because she has been sitting in the chair for too long during the day. One of the main problems here is that Staff Nurse Baker has got into a routine that suits her but is not in line with current best practice. She needs to make some changes.

Through professional regulation, all registered nurses are expected to deliver clinically effective, quality care (NMC, 2008). Evidence-based practice (EBP) requires nurses to be able to find, appraise and, where appropriate, make use of evidence to support their practice. Regarding EBP and learning, the NMC (2004) states that:

> *The development of nursing programmes arises from the premise that nursing is a practice-based profession, recognising the primacy of patient and client well-being and respect for individuals, and is founded on the principles that:*
>
>   *•   evidence should inform practice through the integration of relevant knowledge*
>   *•   students are actively involved in nursing care delivery under supervision*

- *the NMC Code of professional conduct: standards for conduct, performance and ethics applies to all practice interventions*
- *skills and knowledge are transferable*
- *research underpins practice*
- *the importance of lifelong learning and continuing professional development is recognised.*

In this chapter we will define evidence-based practice (EBP), discuss the different types of evidence, including where they might be found, and possible ways to rank that evidence. We will also consider how to use evidence when it requires us to change our practice.

Background

The publication of *The New NHS: Modern, dependable* (DH, 1997) raised widespread awareness of the government's commitment to modernise healthcare provision through the introduction of clinical governance. This was at least, in part, a reaction to serious and occasionally big differences in healthcare delivery. This landmark change of focus in healthcare provision demanded both standardisation and improvement in the quality of all care and treatment. Further publications quickly followed on to reinforce this message, including *A First Class Service* (NHS Executive, 1998), *Saving Lives: Our healthier nation* (DH, 1999a) and *Making a Difference: Strengthening the nursing, midwifery and health visiting contribution to health and healthcare* (DH, 1999b). This latter publication emphasised the crucial role nurses have in working with political plans to modernise the health service and improve public health. In this regard, the government and the NMC are working in partnership, in agreement as to the importance of EBP. A good example of a more recent publication would be the Darzi report, *High Quality for All* (DH, 2008b).

As healthcare professionals, all nurses need to engage with EBP. The NMC (2008) expects nurses to not only act in the client's best interests, but also to deliver care to a quality standard. Morally, nurses should aspire to 'do good' (beneficence) and 'do no harm' (non-maleficence). This should be easier to achieve if sound rationales (sets of reasons) for nursing interventions are available, found, shared and understood.

Since 1997, the government has signposted a long-term commitment to creating an environment in which quality within health and social care is achievable. The Department of Health website describes hundreds of publications that focus on clinical governance and how to achieve quality through the implementation of EBP. On this website you can click through to NHS Evidence, which includes reviews from the Cochrane database (**www.evidence.nhs.uk**).

Within most professions there is sometimes a gap between theory and practice, and this is certainly the case in nursing. When the gap is too wide, it must be formally addressed. The debate continues as to whether it is possible to eradicate the theory–practice gap entirely. In part, this is due to the very different cultural foundations of academic and practical areas. While the NMC does not expect practice to be always in a constant state of change in response to new evidence, where evidence shows that practice needs to develop differently, then it should do so.

Clinical governance requires the delivery of consistently high standards of treatment and care, by healthcare professionals who can engage with all three stages of EBP. EBP is one of the 'pillars' that supports clinical governance. The Care Quality Commission (CQC) is responsible for reviewing the performance of NHS Trusts to make sure that this happens. The National Institute for Health and Clinical Excellence (NICE) is responsible for providing national guidance on how to promote good health and also on the prevention and treatment of ill health. You could view the CQC as an organisation focused on enforcing clinical governance. NICE can be viewed as the 'softer' side of a political process seeking to standardise healthcare quality.

Defining evidence-based practice

Evidence-based practice (EBP) within nursing involves care delivery that is clearly based upon well-considered, applicable evidence that enables, supports and defends effective care. EBP is developed by thoughtful professionals who are committed to improving themselves and their practice in order to deliver good quality care. There is a very real link between healthcare professionals developing their knowledge, skills and attitudes, and working successfully towards delivering better client-centred care.

The process of EBP moves through three fundamental stages (see Figure 8.1). All nurses should be able to search for and find evidence (stage one). The second stage involves critical appraisal, where the quality of the information is evaluated. Once the first two stages of the process are completed, the nurse can be confident about the evidence and defend using it (stage three). This EBP process is part of a quality assurance process that paves the way for effective decision-making.

Fundamentally, there are three main types of academic evidence: primary, original research studies; secondary or integrative work; and tertiary sources, usually offering expert opinion. Let us look in more detail at each type.

Primary sources of evidence

Research is original work that seeks to find out new information and is usually investigative or explorative. The word 'research' refers to the act of looking closer or looking again. Research can fill a gap in knowledge because through the research process we may come to know something that we did not know before. A primary source is like a witness statement: this is evidence that someone has gathered themselves, first-hand. Like a seed, research usually begins with a question, theory or aim; something to develop from. Articulating this aim is a critically important first step towards internal validity. The concept of internal validity basically means that the research methods used must facilitate the research process, from research aim to findings and recommendations, which logically lead to achievement of the aim. We will now look at the various types of primary research.

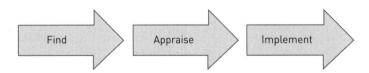

Figure 8.1: The evidence-based practice process

Quantitative research

Quantitative research focuses on developing numerical evidence and often seeks to find evidence for a hypothesis, with an outcome that can be measured. This kind of research uses statistics and numerical analysis. The sample sizes tend to be large so that, in some way, they represent the population being studied. This may be achieved through random selection of participants, where all possible participants have an equal chance of being included. It might require a **stratified sample** where the specific diversity of a sample needs to be represented.

Statistical methods can be used to predict sample sizes large enough to make generalisation from the study to other populations possible and therefore achieving **external validity**. The location, attributes and control of **confounding variables** connected to the sample are critically important in determining whether the research process has proved a theory. For example, if you were comparing wound dressings the comparison would only really be fair if the wounds were similar and being dressed using the same non-touch technique and cleaning solution.

A **randomised controlled trial** is a gold standard quantitative research design in which the measure of success is directly related to the quality of the randomisation and control of confounding variables. These key features establish whether the impact of a new intervention is genuine. This may sound straightforward, but is not always easy. Statistical packages can be used to randomise participants across populations, but controlling the variables that surround live participants can be far more difficult to achieve and maintain over time. Everyone is different and their behaviour is often unpredictable. For example, take the example of comparing wound dressings. A district nurse might be trying out two dressings on similar wounds and one wound does not heal as well. It might be because the dressing does not live up to its promise, but it could be because one patient heals poorly or is even interfering with the wound ('knitting needle syndrome').

Quantitative research provides primary evidence on the effectiveness of an intervention such as a new type of talking therapy, the effectiveness and potential side effects of medication, the success of new wound care treatments or the potency of certain nutritional supplements. For more details on types of quantitative research, see Chapter 5 in Williamson et al. (2008). However, many important aspects of human experience cannot be expressed in numbers, and evidence of this type comes from qualitative research.

Qualitative research

Qualitative research aims to achieve insight into the depth and detail of human experience. This requires equal attention to detail in identifying suitable participants and implementing a clear and defensible research process. So constructing a research design that follows a robust process is just as important as it is in quantitative research, but the methods employed and stated outcomes will invariably be different. Each stage of the research journey may be different, from stated aims, sample choice, methods of data collection and data analysis through to the nature of the findings. Qualitative research may not be able to 'represent' communities or populations, as the sample may be small. Nevertheless, the research can still achieve its aims and therefore achieve internal validity. For more details on types of qualitative research, see Chapter 5 in Williamson et al. (2008).

Once you get used to appraising research, you will need to remember the priority of attending to ethical considerations in all healthcare research. Similar to clinical governance, research governance is concerned with safeguarding the quality of research and protecting the participants involved. This includes achieving the informed consent of participants, assuring confidentiality for them and respecting the voluntary contribution of participants. Fair treatment of all research participants should be achieved and maintained.

The quality of any evidence will depend on how carefully and well it has been designed and put together. No study will be perfect: all research designs have inherent strength and weaknesses. Some studies have a design that strives to achieve insight into both qualitative and quantitative issues, and is called 'mixed method'. This design may appear to increase the complexity of the study, but the critical appraisal of the research should be adapted to ask the right questions of such a complex design.

To be objective, or at least as objective as possible, is a frequently noted aim in the majority of research projects. To attain objectivity, researchers must not be influenced by emotion or prejudice. The phenomena under investigation must be real and independently observable. Within the area of social science research this can be difficult to obtain fully because there are so many variables. Again, the responsibility is upon the researcher(s) to produce a research design that is clear, robust, logically constructed and well defended. The quality of the research can legitimately dictate how influential that evidence is.

Secondary sources of evidence

Secondary sources of evidence are those that review other evidence, often including several comparable pieces of research, with a view to trying to find best evidence through consensus. Secondary sources are often **systematic reviews** or clinical guidelines. Systematic reviews, when they consider gold-standard quantitative evidence, can be regarded as platinum standard because they provide insight into potential consensus across sources of comparable generalisable evidence. A team of reviewers may set inclusion and exclusion criteria and thereafter implement a comprehensive literature search. This may involve not only full database searches, but also hand searches through 'grey publications', appreciating that some very valuable research does not achieve full national publication. It is the completeness of the literature search that defines a systematic review, in conjunction with the quality of the appraisal of that gathered evidence.

Clinical guidelines, particularly national guidelines of the standard produced by the National Institute of Clinical Excellence (NICE) and the Scottish Intercollegiate Guideline Network (SIGN), are similarly a very powerful source. They can be described as a defensible shortcut to high quality accumulation of evidence, which is very useful synthesised information for the busy practitioner. Again, clinical guidelines can be defined by very specific measures of quality in terms of how they have been produced. Clinical guidelines are influenced and informed by the accumulation of information that the guideline development group uncover in its literature searches, which may include a blend of primary, secondary and tertiary evidence. The team can review, appraise and consider this evidence, discussing it in line with their experience. This team effort may very well include consultation with a variety of experts, including service users. Once the guideline group has reviewed the evidence base and reached consensus as to what is defensible best practice, their report needs to be presented in a clear, well-indexed, reader-friendly manner. Ultimately, it needs to be produced and presented in a quality assured way, mindful of its date of publication.

Local policies and procedures are also secondary sources. Although they direct rather than guide practitioners as to the best course of action, they may not have been as robustly constructed. This is concerning because if a statement of established practice is made mandatory, it would be far better to present, inform and support it to a high standard. Considering the very prescriptive nature of working policies, they should be well informed and compliant with national advice as to best practice. To be otherwise potentially puts the accountable healthcare practitioner in a difficult position because Trusts buy indemnity cover to protect themselves. This indemnity cover is only assured by practitioners who practise in accordance with set policies and procedures. Similar to any insurance, the cost is low if the risk is small and the practice is safe. If these policies become outdated (superseded by new information), this can leave the practitioner in a very difficult position.

Secondary sources of evidence can be more time limited than some other sources because of their integrative, reviewing nature. They need a review date for assessing future emerging evidence, and are time limited for up to four years.

Tertiary sources of evidence

Tertiary sources are usually opinions based on the work of experts. As such, they can get 'from idea to print' quite quickly, perhaps within months or even weeks, whereas research generally takes years. Expert opinion may be presented as editorials, briefing papers, opinion-based articles and books. It is more usual for a book to be a tertiary source than any of the other types of evidence. Although their creation may not require the length of time or level of involvement that other sources require, they can make an important contribution to evidence-based practice because they draw on experience and professional opinion. They may be written by academic and professional practitioners who have developed their expertise over many years, putting them in a strong position to offer advice. They should be well presented, supported by literature (referenced) and offer a useful contribution to professional debate on the topic in question.

While tertiary sources can be time limited, each one needs to be assessed on its own merits. They can become seminal works and last for decades – for example, the work of Schön (1987) on reflective practice. However, clinical evidence bases regarding care packages, treatment regimes and specific interventions are superseded when new evidence comes to light. New evidence can challenge practitioners to change, and every practitioner has a responsibility to keep up to date and engage with new ideas when relevant, appropriate and necessary. It is engagement with the process of EBP that reveals when there is the need for change.

When considering the nature of expert opinions, it is important to contemplate what the author's claim to expertise might be. Opinions can be easily offered but also need to be defended.

Evaluating and using evidence

We have considered the features of some examples of different evidence sources. The rigour, clarity and transparency of the process leading to their production are pointers to their quality. Not all sources will have designs that make their results generalisable, or representative beyond the original sample of participants. Most research achieves what it aims to, achieving internal validity. Well-conducted quantitative research, with large representative sample sizes, may also achieve external validity. This is a claim further supported by **transparency of research process**.

Within the medical world, evidence is needed as to whether a treatment is clinically effective across different client groups. Even at this level, where scientific evidence may be generalisable and externally valid across a population, this is still not necessarily straightforward. Let's look at a standard 'classification' of evidence as a starting point from which to consider why evidence may be important to nurses and the people they care for. The concept summary below shows one main interpretation of a hierarchy of evidence. It is important to view the hierarchy of evidence as one interpretation, a starting point for discussion about how we rank evidence in order of importance. What type of evidence is important to you and your order of priorities will depend on your professional perspective. For nurses, who are focused on delivering holistic care, the traditional hierarchy of evidence as shown is up for debate.

Concept summary: an example of a hierarchy of evidence

1. Platinum standard: systematic reviews/multiple randomised controlled trials/**meta-analysis**
2. Gold standard: one well-conducted randomised controlled trial
3. Non-randomised experimental study or equivalent
4. **Non-experimental** quantitative research
5. Clinical guidelines or well-written protocols
6. Qualitative research
7. Expert opinion

It is important to bear in mind that EBP is often better supported by several sources at once, contributing a more powerful 'blend of perspectives' that gain momentum through consensus (agreement).

How to engage with the EBP process

The EBP process often begins for nurses with an uncomfortable feeling of realising there are gaps in their knowledge. For example, if a new sharps disposal system is introduced, you would need to seek out training in how to use it properly. You might also want to find out other practitioners' views on using the new equipment. From this point, it is logical to focus on finding suitable evidence.

Stage 1: Searching for evidence

Having a good level of information literacy skills underpins an effective search for evidence (see Chapter 7 for a more in-depth consideration of this). Information literacy is defined by the ability to identify gaps in knowledge and then formulate a strategy to effectively find current and relevant knowledge, backed by evidence, to address those gaps.

Activity 8.1　　　　　　　　　　　*Evidence-based practice and research*

Look at the databases available through your university library. Which ones do you think would be important for you to use and why? (This issue is considered in some depth in Chapter 7.)

An outline answer is provided at the end of the chapter.

The types of evidence valuable to nursing

The three main types of evidence all have a place within EBP. In fact, it is often the accumulative evidence from several sources that can collectively inform and support changes in practice. However, it is also important to appreciate the differences between these sources, as this can help us to identify when these different types of evidence may be most useful and appropriate to our context or issue.

What you might also find during your searches is that some key authors, who have become experts in their specialist area, may also contribute research, reviews and expert opinions at varying times in their career.

Once you have become familiar with where to look for evidence (often the library, databases and online), how to recognise the different types of sources and thereby gather all the information that you need, the next logical step is to consider the quality of that evidence. This part of the EBP process is called appraisal.

<table>
<tr><td colspan="2"></td></tr>
</table>

Activity 8.2   *Critical thinking*

Constructing a table of source types

On the basis of what we have discussed so far, fill out the following table.

Source type	Main features	Examples	Advantages for nursing practice
Primary sources			
Secondary sources			
Tertiary evidence			

An outline answer is provided at the end of the chapter.

Stage 2: Appraising sources of evidence

For nurses to be truly professional, they need to be independent critical thinkers, capable of demonstrating full accountability upon registration. Just as nurses use the reflection process to be constructively critical of their own and others' practice, they can appraise the quality of any evidence that might be used to inform their practice. The NMC (2010, p4) states that:

> *Our standards aim to enable nurses to give and support high quality care in rapidly changing environments. They reflect how future services are likely to be delivered, acknowledge future public health priorities and address the challenges of long-term conditions, an ageing population, and providing more care outside hospitals. Nurses must be equipped to lead, delegate, supervise and challenge other nurses and healthcare professionals. They must be able to develop practice, and promote and sustain change. As graduates they must be able to think analytically, use problem-solving approaches and evidence in decision-making, keep up with technical advances and meet future expectations.*

Knowing what questions to ask when critically reading evidence is very important. Critical frameworks are useful tools to ask the right questions in the right order to help you make a complete appraisal. Critical frameworks need to match the type of evidence they are used to appraise: you cannot ask the same questions of all sources of evidence.

As discussed earlier in this chapter, primary work is expected to be original and creative, and also well planned and conducted. When appraising such work it is important to consider whether the research aims were achieved, how it was designed and how well it would compare to similar types of research. Keep a good text about research methods close to hand. A small amount of reading around the stated research design may help you to come to a decision about the quality of the paper you are reading, moving beyond describing what is presented in that paper.

P	**PURPOSE of the research:** What is/are the stated aim(s)? This may also be listed in the abstract to a primary source.
R	**RIGOUR of the planning and process:** Was the research carefully planned and then put into place? This may be discussed within the earlier parts of a research article.
I	**INFORMATION sought to inform the research:** Was a literature review included in the research process and when was it completed? In most cases, this would be at the beginning of the article.
M	**MORALITY (ethics), METHODOLOGY (design) and METHODS of data collection (tools):** Were ethical principles adhered to? Did the study have ethical approval? Did the design match the topic? Were the methods of data collection a good fit with the research design?
A	**ANALYSIS of data:** How was the data analysed? Who analysed the data? Were there any efforts made to check understanding from the data with participants?
R	**RESULTS of research:** What was found? What is recommended?
Y	**YEAR of publication:** Is the work still current?

Table 8.1: A critical framework for primary sources

Table 8.1 offers a mnemonic to remind you of the features of research that you should consider when you appraise original work.

Secondary sources of evidence can be very important for busy practitioners because essentially a lot of the hard work has been done within the reviewing process. When well constructed, they can efficiently guide the practitioner to the best courses of action. It is a significant responsibility to offer such synthesised advice and guidance. Therefore, secondary sources need to be well presented, clearly indexed and robustly constructed on the basis of collaborative teamwork.

Table 8.2 presents a mnemonic to remind you of the features of secondary evidence that you should consider when you appraise such work.

Tertiary sources are predominantly referred to as expert opinion. As discussed previously, they tend to be found as books, discussion papers in journals, editorials and briefing papers. Their aim is to inform, raise debate and develop professional understanding.

Table 8.3 offers a mnemonic to remind you of the features of tertiary evidence that you should consider when you appraise such work.

Moving towards applying evidence

The production of any evidence can take time and effort, so it is wasteful when it is not shared, debated and the potential for its use considered. Evidence can be used to improve practice and we can consider this potential through critical reflection. It is often an issue of concern that ignites the reflective process.

S	**SCOPE and purpose of the review:** Who are the guidelines designed for? What is the review being done for? Who will benefit?
E	**EVIDENCE review:** Was a literature review included in the process and when was it completed?
C	**CONSULTANCY and COLLABORATION:** Were service users invited to be involved? Who and how many individual stakeholders were in the review team?
O	**OPENNESS/transparency:** Has the process undertaken in the review/production of the source been made clear?
N	**NEUTRALITY:** Was there any bias evident? Were there any conflicts of interest declared?
D	**DESIGN QUALITY:** Was the process of review robust?
A	**ACCESSIBLITY OF WRITING STYLE:** Is the source well presented? Is the source well indexed with a clear contents list?
R	**RECOMMENDATIONS and REVIEW:** What are the recommendations? Is there a summary of findings?
Y	**YEAR of publication; is there a review date?:** Is the source still current? Is there a stated review date?

Table 8.2: A critical framework for secondary sources

T	**TOPIC relevance:** Is there a clear match between what the source discusses and the topic you are interested in? Is the opinion relevant to your area of practice?
E	**EDITOR and/or peer reviewed:** Has the source been independently reviewed or peer/blind reviewed?
R	**RIGOUR of presentation:** Is the source well presented? Are the arguments clearly signposted? Are there clear sub-headings?
T	**THESIS or argument:** Are the arguments made clearly and well defended?
I	**INFORMATION literacy skills of the author:** Was a literature review included in the process and when was it completed? Is the source well referenced?
A	**AUTHORITY/claim to expertise?:** Who is the author? Are they an acknowledged expert in this area of practice?
R	**RECOMMENDATIONS:** What are the recommendations?
Y	**YEAR of publication:** Is the work still current and/or relevant? Is the source still current?

Table 8.3: A critical framework for tertiary sources

Scenario

Imagine you are a student on the ward with Staff Nurse Baker (who we met on page 154). You have been learning about pressure sores in your skills classes and you know that there are pressure-relieving seat covers for chairs as well as pressure-relieving mattresses for beds. You might be surprised that Staff Nurse Baker has not thought of using such aids. She has talked to you about the risks of lying down too long, but amid her busy routines, often forgets how long clients are sitting up and out of bed.

Activity 8.3   *Critical thinking*

Reflect on the scenario, first by identifying some themes of importance to review. For example, the scenario reveals some issues with the theory–practice gap and how students can come into a clinical area with a fresh perspective. This is not the first time that we have encountered a scenario where someone was shocked or disappointed by what they encountered in practice. In Chapter 9, the issues faced by Staff Nurse Yosef are discussed, when he encounters bad practice during a cardiac arrest. Have a look at that scenario (page 187) and then consider the major themes that you might want to follow up.

A sample answer is provided at the end of the chapter.

Stage 3: Using evidence in practice (implementation phase)

The world of work is complex in nursing as it is in any other profession. As described earlier, there are both professional and political drivers to encourage compliance with evidence-based practice. As it is mandated through NMC regulation, you might expect compliance with EBP to be consistent and well assured in practice. The quality of healthcare is very important for legal, professional and ethical reasons, because of the duty of care, the need to act in the client's best interests and the need to uphold fundamental ethical principles. So there are a myriad of reasons to want practice to be consistently exemplary in its delivery.

However, the progress of any profession is influenced by its own history, issues and limitations. Individual nurses turn up to work with a variety of agendas, attitudes and expectations of themselves. Tradition and authority can maintain poor practice and stop change aimed at improving practice. As you start out on your career pathway in nursing, think about how you can and should want to be an agent for change. The NHS is under constant pressure to be both clinically and cost-effective. This requires smart working by nurses who have the resilience to continue to put clients first in the midst of this complexity. Evidence can also help us to plan for the future. Demographics clearly indicate that we have an ageing population. From this knowledge, we can move towards planning services to meet the needs of older adults.

Stage 3 of EBP is made possible by there being evidence in existence. However, this is not always the case as not all topics are thoroughly researched, reviewed or debated. Evidence also needs to be accessible and of good quality to have the best chance of reaching its target audience. A further issue concerns what we might call non-evidential factors. These are influences that are not in themselves evidence but can affect whether evidence is used or not.

Barriers to evidence-based practice

While not all routines and rituals are bad, if they weaken practitioners' enthusiasm to practise thoughtfully, then they become a problem. If nurses are tired and overworked, they may fear the change that EBP involves. Change can be time and resource consuming and consistently high workloads can dampen enthusiasm.

With so much political, professional and legal pressure on practitioners that promotes compliance with clinical governance and EBP (NMC, 2008), it is timely to explore and identify the barriers working against EBP. From the discussion so far it should be apparent that all three stages of EBP require something of and from the practitioner. Finding evidence is enabled by information literacy skills, but can be time-consuming. Appraisal requires confidence, can also be very time consuming, and some peer-reviewed journal articles can be hard to interpret and understand. Both of these stages could be developed on a small scale by individuals, but knowledge and understanding of the processes involved needs to be developed. However, the implementation stage is far more likely to require a team effort.

Nurses are working practitioners, often with a very full clinical workload, in an environment where there are often nursing shortages and little chance of short-term improvements in staffing levels despite increasingly acute clinical demands. EBP is a high expectation of overworked and under-resourced practitioners. Challenge and change that develops professional work practice operates within a social and cultural context, and this can present barriers to the extra workload EBP brings with it. Yet professional status often requires 'going the extra mile', so what are the potential solutions?

Enablers of evidence-based practice

Like the establishment of clinical governance generally, the implementation of EBP is made possible by professional enthusiasm about change when change is required as well as organisational commitment. Practitioners can be at the forefront of recognising when change is necessary. Individual nurses can make a difference by noticing that there is a problem and making change themselves. Take, for example, the 'red tray system' that was used in several hospitals as an immediate visual cue to highlight patients at risk of malnutrition. This simple yet effective innovation made a positive difference to this aspect of patient care. As time and most resources are finite, EBP may involve reorganising priorities and recognising the capacity to engage in new working practices. EBP is often focused on change in the short to medium term, so while evidence might offer choices it must have fundamental goal(s) in mind, usually aimed at improving practice quite quickly. A further example of this would be wall-mounted individual medicine lockers next to patients' beds. There is an initial cost, but thereafter there may be very real benefits for safe drug administration and infection control.

The implementation stage of EBP is forward looking, with awareness of the need for the change and a clear plan. The rationale for the change (reason to believe there will be potential benefits) and some rudimentary ideas as to how (project planning), where and what that change may involve are therefore essential. These features are the fundamental building blocks of organisational change management, which usually requires a well-informed team effort. We might compare this process with the nursing process. The need for change needs to be established through assessment of practice at the time – this might uncover a knowledge gap. The rationale for offering daily mouth care is a classic example. If practice is not as good as required, then the case for change emerges. The response to that need must be carefully planned in order to set out how it can be achieved. Potential costs, such as toothbrushes, need to be factored in. Progress can then be evaluated to consider whether the change has been effective or not. Patient evaluation forms, like satisfaction surveys, might be useful. This underpins the type of quality assurance process that can make EBP a creative reality.

As much as individual participation and engagement is important, so is a degree of organisational commitment to the change process. Goodman and Clemow (2008) discuss issues related to nursing and working with other professional groups. This important consideration is vital in contemplating how the need for change can be managed by and between professional groups. The Darzi report (2008b) includes discussion about why and how this should happen, through better working partnerships and integration of services.

Exploring and integrating the various 'ways of knowing' in nursing can reveal and advance the development of nursing competence and potentially expertise (Benner, 1984). This may demonstrate the value of the many (or at least four) ways of knowing within nursing (Carper, 1978), which include empirical or technical knowledge, aesthetic knowing or the art of nursing, personal understanding and ethical awareness (as later extended and applied by Johns' reflective model, see page 184). Such an approach values the complexity and diversity of nursing knowledge. Nurses need EBP but they can also sometimes harness the potential of their intuition, not least because they are the client's advocate.

Service user and carer involvement

Within the Standards for Pre-registration Nursing Education, the NMC (2010, p113) state that:

> *People can trust the newly registered graduate nurse to treat them as partners and work with them to make a holistic and systematic assessment of their needs; to develop a personalised plan that is based on mutual understanding and respect for their individual situation promoting health and well-being, minimising risk of harm and promoting their safety at all times.*

Service user and carer involvement is an essential component of EBP. It is critically important that any consumer of healthcare, wherever possible, is encouraged to feel involved, consulted and responded to. There are a variety of levels at which service users want to engage with EBP. Every individual who accepts treatment or care from any healthcare practitioner is putting their trust in them to deliver effective care on the basis of sound knowledge and defensible evidence. Professional status and clinical governance really demand that such expectations are met. However, delivering clinically effective healthcare packages is largely dependent on having well-supported resources in place. Nurses have a central co-ordinating role and should aspire to be effective advocates for their clients. These responsibilities mean that you are often a central point of liaison between service users, informal carer and other health and social care practitioners. EBP is often about identifying best practice, but could also be a springboard to considered treatment and care options, all of which might be clinically effective to varying degrees. The service user can be proactive, well informed and assertive enough to challenge poor or sub-optimal practice, when they encounter it. Clinical governance has progressed with service user involvement as a central expectation. Information to inform, or in some cases misinform, service users is often freely available and they have every right to challenge decisions made for them. Access to free information via district libraries and the internet has contributed to raising client expectations of standards of care.

Scenario

Brian is a user of mental healthcare services and he is being introduced to one of the new talking therapies involving cognitive behavioural therapy. He wants reassurance that his existing anti-depressant medication will continue and that he will be regularly consulted as to whether the new intervention is making a distinct difference for him. As he has been invited to take part in a clinical trial to study this new combined treatment, he will want not only to feel involved, but also truly listened to when he offers feedback on his experiences.

No one intervention will suit everyone. There will be some service users for whom the side effects of some medications or treatments are so unpleasant that the benefit of the drug is outweighed by the adverse effects of taking it. So service user involvement is also important in terms of challenging standardised practice, even when it might be considered clinically effective best practice. Where appropriate, it adds another voice of support to try to make evidence-based practice a reality. All service users have fundamental human rights and the Mental Capacity Act (Department of Health, 2005) reinforces that. Nurses need to ensure informed consent by clearly presenting their assessments and plans to service users, listening to their responses and, if necessary, advocating for choice rather than presenting one clinically effective option. Collaborative working with service users and, where appropriate, their carers completes the picture of the essential components of EBP, as shown in Figure 8.2. Note that the service user is shown in the centre of the figure. This is a deliberate reminder that one of the most important features of clinical governance is that the service user is situated at the centre of their care package.

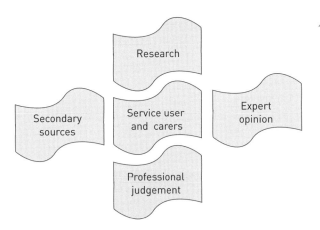

Conclusion

The landscape of evidence-based practice is strengthened not just by consensus of evidence but also by its diversity, especially considering the needs of service users. Ethically, this must involve consumers at whatever level they feel comfortable because it is to them that healthcare needs to be delivered and they have rights. There needs to be a balance between theory presented (within or beyond the classroom) and practical skills acquisition (predominantly gained within practice) because professional nursing needs both. However, effective ongoing dialogue between theory and practice is vital because the tension between them offers opportunities for constructive change and development.

Chapter summary

Within this chapter we have reviewed what EBP is, what the stages of EBP are, what sources of evidence might inform EBP and how we might rank them. Some new critiquing tools have been suggested, with consideration of their structure. How nurses might progress through the three main stages of EBP has been considered, and the barriers and enablers of change have been discussed. This has been presented within a social and political context in which clinical governance is a reality and the expectation of the NMC is that nurses deliver client-centred EBP.

Activities: Brief outline answers

Activity 8.1 (page 161)

The main nursing databases currently on offer include the Cumulative Index for Nurses and Allied Health Professionals (CINAHL) and the British Nursing Index (BNI). These are highly relevant and will often be the first places that nurses search for evidence. CINAHL is a large database of international journals, which offers sophisticated advanced searching options presented online. BNI is a much smaller database but offers more local journal articles. It does not have the same level of search options. Any defensible search for nursing literature should involve both databases. In addition, depending on the topic to be considered, other databases including Medline (mostly medical evidence/articles), PsychInfo (including mental health evidence) and the Cochrane Collaboration (a storehouse of high quality systematic reviews), may offer additional range and depth to the literature search.

Activity 8.2 (page 162)

Here are some suggestions, but you may have identified even more.

Source type	Main features	Examples	Advantages for nursing practice
Primary sources	Methods, methodology, ethics, original, creates new knowledge	Randomised controlled trial Case control Survey Qualitative research Grounded theory	Offers new knowledge Scientific credibility Can be practitioner led
Secondary sources	Integrative Evaluative Retrospective Collaborative Consultative Short-lived	Systematic reviews Meta-analysis Clinical guidelines	Can reveal consensus regarding best practice Defensible shortcut to synthesised evidence
Tertiary evidence	Opinion based Often referenced Contributes to professional debate	Journal articles Briefing papers Editorials Books Continuing education papers	Raises issues in the press quickly Often respects experience Often very accessible

Activity 8.3 (page 165)

While there are many themes that could be drawn from the scenario, there are two that I picked up on.

1 What is the last sense to go?

While there might be some professional scepticism as to whether any senses can be 'active' when an individual is in cardiac arrest, Parnia et al. (2007) discuss some anecdotal evidence that indicates that hearing might be possible. They cite near-death experiences and accounts of 'out-of-body' experiences that challenge our thinking. They discuss some of the tensions and challenges in trying to research such a topic, including how you would recruit research participants. They state that:

> Using what is understood from awareness during anaesthesia it may thus be possible to conclude that perhaps during cardiac arrest there are different levels of consciousness depending on the degree of cerebral depression which occurs as a consequence of reduced cerebral blood flow. However, much of the evidence regarding cerebral function during cardiac arrest indicates that there is a lack of electrical activity in the brain during cardiac arrest.
> (Parnia et al., 2007, p218)

So Staff Nurse Yosef is right to feel concerned, because it is possible that the patient might have heard the unfortunate comments from the senior nurse.

2 Why are nurses sometimes unsupportive towards new staff?

The social processes or occupational socialisation underpinning practice are recognised as an established phenomenon within many professions. Occupational socialisation, with associated effects upon student learning, is a real and enduring issue in clinical practice, with far-reaching consequences (Whitcombe, 2005).

Through this social process the student may internalise how to work within the healthcare team. This participation may operate at the level of compliance where students may endeavour to fit in with 'normal' practices and role modelling (Clouder, 2004; Spouse, 2000). This may not impact on their internal beliefs leading to full conformity but rather demonstrate a pragmatic approach to temporary participation within the clinical environment (Clouder, 2004; Spouse, 2000).

This arguably demonstrates a strategic individual response to an awareness of the vulnerable status of the temporary participant. This involves 'learning how to play the game' as Melia (1987) described. *The possibility of strategic compliance therefore reinforces scepticism that novice professionals simply accommodate to expectations* (Clouder, 2003, p215). Beyond this there is the possibility that particularly the young and inexperienced novice truly conforms and is actually transformed by the experience in terms of beliefs as well as behaviours, rather than temporarily 'bending to the rules'.

Further reading

Ellis, P (2010) *Evidence-based Practice in Nursing.* Exeter: Learning Matters.

Ellis, P (2010) *Understanding Research for Nursing Students.* Exeter: Learning Matters.

Whittaker, A and Williamson, GR (2011) *Succeeding in Research Project Plans and Literature Reviews for Nursing Students.* Exeter: Learning Matters.

These books in the 'Transforming Nursing Practice' series look at EBP and research in more detail.

Fitzpatrick, J (2007) Finding the research for evidence-based practice, Part One. *Nursing Times*, 103 (19): 32–3.

Fitzpatrick, J (2007) Finding the research for evidence-based practice, Part Two: Selecting credible evidence. *Nursing Times*, 103 (17): 32–3. Available online at www.nursingtimes.net

Fitzpatrick, J (2007) How to turn research into evidence-based practice, Part Three: Making a case. *Nursing Times*, 103 (19): 32–3.

A useful series of articles from a subject matter expert and regular teacher in EBP.

Gray, A and Harrison, S (2004) *Governing Medicine, Theory and Practice.* Berkshire: Open University Press.

A very insightful text discussing the rationale, history and progress of clinical governance.

Useful websites

www.agreecollaboration.org/instrument

Here you will find the full appraisal tool for guidelines, with additional information on how to make use of it.

www.badscience.net

A fascinating website where Ben Goldacre reviews various sources of questionable evidence, which he very ably critiques and challenges.

www.cqc.org.uk

The official website of the Care Quality Commission (CQC).

www.dh.gov.uk

The official website of the Department of Health, where you will find a list of its publications.

www.evidence.nhs.uk

A clinically focused collection of evidence.

www.nelm.nhs.uk/en/Categories/National-Health

This site provides key information including medicines by name, guidelines and clinical governance updates.

www.nice.org.uk

The official website of the National Institute of Clinical Excellence (NICE), which includes a list of its publications.

www.sign.ac.uk

The official website of the Scottish Intercollegiate Guideline Network (SIGN), which includes a list of its publications.

Chapter 9
Reflection: looking backwards, moving forwards

Nicola Davis

NMC Standards for Pre-registration Nursing Education

This chapter will address the following competencies:

Domain 1: Professional values

7. All nurses must be responsible and accountable for keeping their knowledge and skills up to date through continuing professional development. They must aim to improve their performance and enhance the safety and quality of care through evaluation, supervision and appraisal.
8. All nurses must practise independently, recognising the limits of their competence and knowledge. They must reflect on these limits and seek advice from, or refer to, other professionals where necessary.

Domain 4: Leadership, management and team working

4. All nurses must be self-aware and recognise how their own values, principles and assumptions may affect their practice. They must maintain their own personal and professional development, learning from experience, through supervision, feedback, reflection and evaluation.

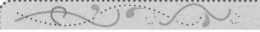
NMC Essential Skills Clusters

This chapter will address the following ESCs:

Cluster: Care, compassion and communication

1. As partners in the care process, people can trust a newly registered graduate nurse to provide collaborative care based on the highest standards, knowledge and competence.

5. People can trust the newly registered graduate nurse to engage with them in a warm, sensitive and compassionate way.

By entry to the register

13. Through reflection and evaluation demonstrates commitment to personal and professional development and life-long learning.

continued overleaf . . .

continued . . .

Cluster: Organisational aspects of care

12. People can trust the newly registered graduate nurse to respond to their feedback and a wide range of other sources to learn, develop and improve services.

By the second progression point:

3. Uses supervision and other forms of reflective learning to make effective use of feedback.

14. People can trust the newly registered graduate nurse to be an autonomous and confident member of the multi-disciplinary or multi agency team and to inspire confidence in others.

By the second progression point:

4. Reflects on own practice and discusses issues with other members of the team to enhance learning.

Chapter aims

By the end of this chapter, you should be able to:

- demonstrate a fundamental understanding of what reflective practice is;
- recognise some straightforward models designed to structure reflection;
- understand how reflection can help develop your practice;
- be prepared to start writing reflective accounts.

Introduction

In this chapter we will consider how you can really capitalise on the learning opportunities all around you. You might not realise it, but we are learning from experience all the time. Reflection can bring that learning to the surface, making us more conscious of what is going on around us. This may extend the opportunities to learn effectively from that experience, through to developing new knowledge and skills.

Reflection involves thinking critically about experiences that you have had, or are currently undergoing, and considering how you can learn effectively from them. This is important because as you prepare to become a nurse or midwife, you are working towards professional practice and professionals are expected to aspire to improve as they establish themselves within their work. The NMC (2008d) expects all practitioners registered with them to engage in continuous professional development (CPD) as working professionals, as indicated by the statements made within Domain 4. This CPD includes learning throughout your working career (lifelong learning), engaging with evidence-based practice (seeking to improve) and reflecting on your practice (practising thoughtfully). Reflection, while not always a comfortable experience, should help you recognise, review, explore and therefore capitalise on your experiential learning. Within this chapter, we will consider further what reflection is, and look at two main types of reflection. We will also look at the benefits of reflection and at some models that offer various approaches to making reflection work for you through a structured process.

The reflective skills you develop may well improve your ability to recall, describe and document your experiences. By analysing these experiences, you will develop your intellectual skills and increase your self-awareness: assessing your strengths, weaknesses, learning needs and opportunities.

Scenario

Grace is a year-one nursing student starting her first practice learning opportunity. When she goes on to the ward on the first day, she joins the team in the handover. Within the first few minutes it is clear to Grace that she cannot understand most of what is being said because there is too much jargon. She is too nervous to ask for explanations, and comes out of the handover unsure of what to do next.

This could be viewed as quite a challenging situation – a potential barrier – but it could also be seen as a learning opportunity. Grace is enthusiastic to find out what the jargon means and why it is used. She starts reflecting on why this problem has arisen and who might be able to help her. We will return to Grace's story later and consider some possible solutions.

What is reflection?

For you, as a student, reflection is a valuable strategy in exploring practice encounters whether you are alone, with peers in enquiry-based learning or even in preparation for formal assessments of your knowledge and understanding. Reflection underpins good professional practice because it provides opportunities to review current practice and identify areas that you need to develop further. It is an ongoing, dynamic process, one in which you can be often engaged. It should feel challenging but not overwhelming. Reflection can also help you identify those areas of practice you have already successfully developed. In this case, there may be opportunities to think about how you can share this information with other practitioners, perhaps by feeding back at a meeting, creating a poster to be displayed for peers or writing an article to submit for publication. Your peers can learn with you as you explore issues related to your practice. Later on, you might refer to that as group supervision or action learning.

Reflection at its simplest can be seen as an internal process through which you reconsider what you are doing, and thereby achieve a better awareness of what informs and influences your practice. It is one key way in which professionals carefully consider and develop themselves (Schön, 1987). Some theorists may suggest that reflection starts with an uncomfortable feeling. That might be because an area of practice does not 'seem right', but it might just be that you sense that this is an area that you need to know more about. Almost inevitably, this will begin with a period of contemplation and description of what happened, to set the context. This needs to be carefully reviewed in order for you to move forward to future challenge and change in practice.

There are two main types of reflection, and which one you adopt may depend on your individual learning preferences. They are:

- reflection-on-action;
- reflection-in-action.

Reflection-on-action is as a retrospective activity in which you look back on and evaluate current skills, competencies, knowledge and professional practice.

> ### Scenario
>
> *Abraham is worried about his lack of wound care experience now that he is out in the community on practice learning experience in a local Primary Care Trust. He wants to get the most out of the working relationship he is building up with his new mentor. He senses that his mentor will be more motivated to share her knowledge with him if he is prepared with some background knowledge and asks some relevant questions. He decides to go to the university library and find some relevant articles on leg ulcer assessment and compression bandaging.*

The NMC standards are overtly concerned with all of the attributes enabling effective nursing practice. Several of the established reflective models can guide and structure reflection-on-action, an activity that is best recorded in note or essay form, and therefore capitalised on by writing up these accounts. Alternatively, reflection-in-action can be seen as a more dynamic process of considering current professional practice as it occurs, and developing a deeper understanding of it.

> ### Scenario
>
> *Year-three student Katrin is finding it hard to ask the support staff to help her because she does not feel empowered to do so. She feels her position is one of being delegated to, yet she knows that she must work towards learning how to delegate herself. As Katrin works in the department, she starts to reflect on how she is communicating with staff. She asks herself how can she achieve that fine balance between co-operative working and the appropriate exercise of authority when co-ordinating teamwork?*

Reflection-in-action can challenge you during your working experiences, causing you to reconsider how you can react and make decisions in practice. This is predominantly an internal process, which does not make it any less important, just harder to recall over time.

Distinctions between different types of reflection may seem unclear at times, but that is not the fundamentally important issue. What matters is the process of reflective activity itself, which is of more importance than the individual strategy you use to make it happen. There are many ways to make reflection work for you, including options for structuring reflection. All of these options are acceptable within the broad landscape of reflective practice, as long as you sense a benefit to your practice. The experience may not always be pleasant, but the learning outcome should ideally be productive.

The value of reflection

Reflection becomes the basis for history, the present, and the future. If people do not consider the events of their past, they are unable to take advantage of their present and powerless to shape their future . . .
(Taylor, 2006, p17).

Taylor states precisely why you need to reflect on your practice. You need to be as enthusiastic about your career and its development for as long as you are in nursing, not just at the beginning. Your career will develop and you will change, as nursing itself will change. You need to be able to adapt, achieve job satisfaction and offer a quality service to the people you care for. Before we go on to explore these points, look at Activity 9.1 below. Think about your experience of the possible value reflection has had for you so far. Some possible positive outcomes might be the capacity to share ideas and stories and to 'think aloud'. Sharing stories with a view to learning from them and exchanging ideas often underpins problem-based learning, which may be used as a forum to ignite interest, motivate learning or even assess your advancing knowledge and understanding.

Activity 9.1   *Communication*

Discuss with some of your peers whether you already consider your practice in a reflective way, either during your shifts on placement or after them. If you haven't yet been on placement, ask someone who has, perhaps another student at a different stage in the programme. What are the benefits, and challenges, involved with thinking in this way?

As this is based on your own experiences, there is no outline answer provided.

The activity may have triggered quite a few discussion points for you – some positive, some perhaps more challenging. For example, you may have found that reflection allowed you to think of a solution to a problem you had not recognised at the time, which will be useful to you next time you are faced with a similar experience because you may thereafter react differently. Alternatively, it may have made you interested and excited about an aspect of nursing that is new to you and made you want to find out more.

Reflection should be an enlightening and empowering process that helps accelerate your learning and therefore your development. Possible challenges to considering your practice in a reflective way may include lack of time, pressure of workload and lack of knowledge or confidence about how to think reflectively. Sometimes reflecting can be difficult or even anxiety-provoking, especially when reflecting on events that have not gone well. We will return to these challenges later in the chapter.

Activity 9.2   *Communication*

If you have already been on a placement the scenario involving Grace at the beginning of this chapter (page 175) may have very real resonance for you. Thinking back to that

continued overleaf . . .

---

continued . . .

vignette, what justification can you think of for the use of jargon in handovers? What could Grace do to feel more comfortable when faced with such language at future handovers?

An outline answer is provided at the end of the chapter.

Having considered whether you already engage in some reflective practice, you might want to consider how reflection could positively impact on your future personal development. The reason for the reflective approach is mostly connected to the way you can capitalise on experience as a learning opportunity, helping your understanding of practice. This can involve identifying gaps in knowledge, and therefore searching for new knowledge, and considering theoretical justifications and rationales for practical action. Carper's (1978) work is particularly interesting in this context, because it reminds us that within professional nursing practice we have the opportunity to consider several streams of information and experience, all of which can inform and influence our work. This includes appreciating our personal values, current evidence, ethics and even, where appropriate, our intuition.

Since 1997, the Department of Health has, little by little, advanced its expectations regarding practitioner engagement with clinical governance, focusing on the importance of achieving standardised levels of quality care. One of the major positives of reflection is that it can energise your engagement with the quality agenda. As you would expect, the NMC reiterates these expectations of evidence-based practice and service user involvement, expectations that may occasionally sit at odds with each other. Reflection can be very important in helping you to think through your personal and ethical beliefs, helping you to unpick the effects such beliefs have in the workplace.

Modes of reflection

In the last section we considered the general value of reflection. We can now extend the discussion from contemplating *why* we reflect to *how* we can do it. Taylor (2006) describes three types of reflection: technical, practical and emancipatory.

Technical reflection

This type of reflection considers the theoretical underpinning of practice and forms an important component of achieving evidence-based practice – for example, considering the evidence base underpinning certain types of talking therapies such as Cognitive Behavioural Therapy or Motivational Interviewing. This type of reflection shows that there can be a very pragmatic function to reflection, reaching more in-depth explanation of interactions and interpretation of events, and finding some evidence to defend your practice.

Practical reflection

This involves considering and critiquing current social contexts and interactions, and imagining how such dynamic relationships can be improved. For example, practical reflection might consider the barriers to interprofessional working (such as shortages of time and staff) and consider strategies to overcome them.

Emancipatory reflection

This involves perhaps one of the most potentially satisfying reasons to engage in reflection, that of challenging existing assumptions, rituals and routine, and through doing so, potentially trans-forming practice. To emancipate means to set free, so emancipatory reflection should free you from something holding your practice back. For example, it might challenge the organisational driving forces that often lead to a patient being kept nil-by-mouth for excessive periods of time while theatre lists are managed. In doing so, the driving force might change from organisational expediency to genuine service-user centred care. It is important to realise the potential for passionate and well-informed healthcare practitioners to contribute as change makers, auditing, evaluating and developing practice. This emancipatory function enables practitioners to achieve a consideration of their practice that is in-depth, cathartic and enabling. Everything will be done the way it has always been done until someone sees a better way of doing it and makes the change happen. Traditions sometimes need to be challenged.

So the achievements of reflection can be practical (challenging existing ways of working), psycho-dynamic (defusing and working through inter-agency stress and tensions) or creative (considering new ways of working). All of these approaches are equally legitimate and all are enhanced by a constructive questioning approach. It involves critical thinking, challenging your thoughts, understanding relevant theory and assessing the quality of these sources of knowledge. We will consider critical thinking now in more depth.

Critical thinking

Taylor (2006) states that:

> *Humans have the potential to think, and to think about thinking, because we are endowed with the gifts of memory and reflection. When we take time to reflect, we allow ourselves to attune to deeper levels of awareness, even if only in momentary flashes, as we raise thoughts to consciousness.*
> (Taylor, 2006, p7).

Critical thinking can also be referred to as reflective thinking (Edwards, 1998), underpinning thought-ful practice. This reflective thinking is facilitated by a tolerance for ambiguity rather than a focus on simple problem solving (Jones and Brown, 1991). This is important for you to consider as you start to develop your problem-solving and decision-making skills. This approach can help you start to understand the complexity of practice, and how you can learn from it and adapt appropriately to it.

With practice, you will be able to move forward with your reflection until ultimately you will be able to engage with critical thinking or reasoning. As Bandman and Bandman (1995) put it:

> *reasoning [is that with] . . . which we analyse the use of language, formulate problems, clarify and explicate assumptions, weigh evidence, evaluate conclusions, discriminate between good and bad arguments and seek to justify those facts that result in credible beliefs and actions.*
> (Bandman and Bandman,1995, p7).

Making time for reflective practice

The discussion within this chapter so far may make you feel as though reflective practice is quite a complex and time-consuming activity. You might already have begun to appreciate how busy the nursing role can be, even while you are preparing for it. So it might seem as if there is very little time to engage in reflective activity, during or even after practice.

Think back to Activity 9.1 (page 177). Did that exploration of your practice in a reflective way include considering lack of time and pressure of workloads? It is a good idea to make conscious decisions about when to reflect amid a busy and diverse workload, either by looking at your actions as you work (reflecting *in* practice), or by aiming to reflect later (reflecting *on* practice). Any busy healthcare professional may have to aim somewhere between these two main types of reflection but nevertheless be actively involved in lifelong learning and evidence-based practice.

It is therefore important to recognise that the process of reflection need not be inevitably time-consuming or intrusive on day-to-day practice. Nevertheless, reflective practice requires a variety of skills, some of which we have already touched on, and the need for such skills might be viewed as a barrier. But engaging in reflective activity can be as straightforward or complicated as you would like it to be. The skills that could potentially be involved in reflective activity therefore need to be unpacked and demystified.

Learning from experience

An essential attribute of reflective practice is its capacity to reveal and enhance opportunities for you to learn from practical experience. Learning from experience is a very important part of adult education and involves being both thoughtful and constructively critical about scenarios encountered within practice, perhaps reflecting upon your own performance and that of others. A key thinker on reflection, Schön (1983) suggested that sometimes practitioners only engage in superficial problem solving, which leaves them more likely just to conform to practical routines under pressure of work in a relatively unquestioning manner. This might be understandable under certain circumstances, but as we discussed earlier, technical reflection can have a very real benefit in terms of identifying areas of practice that are defensible and therefore compliant with clinical governance. Alternatively, in some situations we can engage in more critical reflection, considering in more depth how defensible current practice is and where it might appear timely to contemplate change.

Self-awareness and descriptive skills

If the first stage of reflection involves description, then we can also enhance that process by being more faithful narrators of stories, both to ourselves and others. The relevant reflective skills in this context include the ability to accurately recall what happened. This involves being timely, keeping track of the story (to avoid hindsight bias) and being self-aware of your performance. Be aware of yourself as you work: notice the time, what people say and where things are. Nurses make good witnesses because they can notice detail and remember well. Accurate recall is probably the first thing you need to develop when starting to reflect on your practice, as the process of reflection starts with describing that story. It also involves the skill of being able, then to describe practice as it has been experienced.

Seeing evidence and developing evaluative skills

Reflective skills include the ability to constructively evaluate sources of evidence that potentially influence a situation on which you are reflecting. Is the information first-hand? Did you see and hear the event yourself or is this 'knowledge' based on hearsay (or gossip)? This indicates that it is useful to integrate an evidence-based process within the reflective process. However, it is essential to be able to locate sources of evidence first, which is something we considered in depth in Chapter 7.

Analytical skills

Moving beyond description is vital to make the most of our capacity to raise challenge and effect change. Reflective skills should therefore include the ability to analyse an experience and truly understand its importance. Analysis is a core intellectual skill involving critical thinking. To analyse means to break down an issue or problem, and involves looking closely for micro-issues, specific themes and issues of significance within the scenario. This is a similar approach to critical appraisal, which we considered in Chapter 8, and will also be considering later within this chapter.

Application skills

As previously discussed (see page 155), you may feel there is a gap between theory and practice. How do you apply and share what you already know and the information that is accessible to you? Reflective skills can inform, empower and therefore facilitate your ability to make this jump across the gap between theory and practice. They will help you achieve something useful with your new-found knowledge and insight. This process can be simplified and shared, and group reflection can help towards this and overcome some of the perceived barriers to reflection, such as resistant attitudes, through co-operative team effort. Within group reflection, individuals can interpret the experiences of others and identify with them, as they may have experienced similar situations within their own practice. This can be an opportunity to think about the depth and range of nursing practice and the scope of professional practice. Even working within identified policies and procedures, there can still be a safe range of practice and it is possible for qualified practitioners to perform competently with different levels of knowledge and experience. You could explore this with your peers within enquiry-based learning opportunities, because healthcare professionals need to be able to offer clients choices, working in partnership with them.

Models designed to facilitate reflection

To start reflecting using all of the above skills might seem like a big challenge. As with any journey, you might consider using a map. A model of reflection can offer you a conceptual map or guide to structure the progress of your learning journey. There are a variety of reflective models available and they all have some positive design features. It is very much a matter of individual preference whether you always use a particular model or whether you try each of them at different times.

A model is designed to represent, structure and therefore facilitate understanding. Models for reflection can help to simplify, structure and develop the process of reflection. We will examine some key examples of the different models currently available within this chapter.

A model may help to initiate and encourage reflective practice by prompting your thoughts, particularly when you are just getting used to reflecting. This need not constrain the range and potential complexity of reflection, especially as you become more accomplished at working in this way. There are several models of reflection to structure the reflective activity available. You might decide that you do not want to work within an established model of reflection and may wish to construct your own. Where you are learning, there may already be a preferred model, and it is worth finding out what this is. Either way, it is useful to consider a representative selection of these models, considering both structure and content, as you may come across a range of them when you are doing some further reading into this subject.

The models we will look at in this chapter are Driscoll's model, Gibbs' reflective cycle, Johns' model and the Davis model.

Driscoll's model

This is probably the easiest model to start with. It does have more complex versions (Driscoll, 2007), a very good example of which is listed in the Further reading section at the end of this chapter. However at its most simple it comprises three questions: What, So what, and Now what? (see Figure 9.1).

Look very carefully at these three fundamental questions, which form a secure foundation from which to progress your reflections.

- *What?*
  This can be seen as the description stage. You may recall we considered the need to be able accurately to recall stories from practice in a timely manner, with a view to learning from them.
- *So what?*
  This question is asking you to consider why this story or issue is important to you: what makes it so meaningful? Answering this question can involve the analytical and evaluation skills we mentioned earlier.
- *Now what?*
  This question prompts the action stage, where you can contemplate how practice might be different in the future. Answering this question involves the application skills we mentioned earlier.

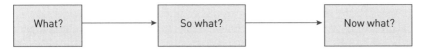

Figure 9.1: Driscoll's model of reflection
Source: Driscoll and Teh (2001)

Driscoll's model is therefore asking you to recall what it is that you want to reflect on, consider why this issue is important and then to contemplate what could be different. Even within this very simple representation, this model covers some of the most important facets of a reflective process.

Consider the case of Grace again. Her story started with feeling uncomfortable in handover because she did not understand much of what was being said and yet knew that the handover was an important part of the information-sharing process between staff. It was important because initially she would need the information in order to be able to contribute to the team effort of caring for the patients on the ward. Later on, Grace will have to learn how to give handovers. In order to prepare for that time, she knows that she needs the help of her mentor in order to acquire the appropriate knowledge and skills.

Gibbs' model

Gibbs' model of reflective practice is a cyclical model. As such, it represents the ongoing and dynamic nature of reflection and visualises the idea that it is an active process. As with most reflective models, this model starts with description, revealing the context of the narrative, and then encourages consideration of the emotions involved and why this narrative is important.

While engaging with this process, you can then break the story down into themes of importance, analyse the features of the case and finally, perhaps most importantly, contemplate whether change is necessary and possible. As with most cyclical processes, the reflection may 'spill over' into another cycle, especially if the scenario is particularly complex or occurs over a long period of time. Figure 9.2 shows the core features of this model.

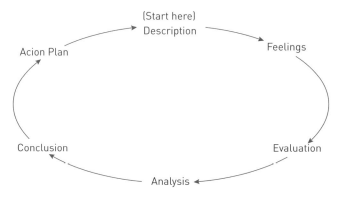

Figure 9.2:
Gibbs' model of reflective practice.
Source: Gibbs (1988)

Activity 9.3	*Decision-making*

Let's consider the dilemma faced by Jo-Yan, a nursing student who has always had a fear of injections. She is worried that she will not be able to cope with giving injections and is frightened to ask her mentor for advice. The emotional impact of this scenario is that Jo-Yan feels more and more anxious and nervous as the placement progresses. Who or what could help her? Could there be a potential change for the better here?

An outline answer is provided at the end of the chapter.

Johns' model

Johns' model is a linear model of questions to guide reflection. It is influenced by Carper's theory regarding what she terms 'ways of knowing' (Carper, 1978). Johns' (1996, 2004) model offers a viable alternative to other models such as those described above. Johns has continued to develop his model of structured reflection, appreciating the varied aspects of knowledge that influence the development of nurses. It provides an important learning opportunity because the complexity of healthcare practice can be informed by many streams of information, which are listed in the model, shown in Table 9.1. Depending on your preferences and perspective, you might like this

Write a description of the experience. **Cue questions**	
Aesthetics Appreciating the artistry underpinning practice, e.g. intuition	• What was I trying to achieve? • Why did I respond as I did? • What were the consequences of that for the patient, others or me? • How was this person/were these people feeling? • How did I know this?
Personal knowing Considering the emotional perspective	• How did I feel in this situation? • What internal factors were influencing me?
Ethics Considering the moral perspective	• How did my actions match with my beliefs? • What factors made me act in incongruent ways?
Empirics Appreciating the scientific knowledge underpinning practice, e.g. research, theory	• What knowledge informed me or should have informed me?
Reflexivity Contemplating the capacity for reflective action, informed by the past, yet focused on the future	• How does this connect with previous experience? • Could I handle this better in similar situations? • What would be the consequences of alternative action for the patient, others or myself? • How do I feel about the experience? • Can I support others and myself better as a consequence? • Has this changed my ways of knowing?

Table 9.1: Johns' model of structured reflection (version 10)

model better. At first glance, you can see it has more questions and they are more detailed. There are indeed several complicated interpretations of this model. It is potentially a more prescriptive and linear approach, which might frame the completeness of your reflections better, particularly as you are starting to work in this way when you record your stories from practice in a portfolio or reflective journal. This model is well suited to guide the production of a written reflective account.

This model does ask a lot of questions and you may find the length of it challenging. However, it is important to look at the types of questions being asked and consider why these headings have been used. This model is important because it reminds us that there are several different streams of information that influence our practice. Using such a highly structured model may be very helpful in unpacking those different influences as you start to work this way in practice, which could ultimately lead to a lengthy and detailed written reflection.

Case study: An example using Johns' model

Description: Lucy is a first-year student working an early shift with her mentor and is asked to take a patient's observations. Lucy goes to the store cupboard and collects an electronic vital signs monitoring device. Her mentor finds her half-way through taking all the patient's observations and tells her to put the machine back and get the manual sphygmomanometer and stethoscope instead. Lucy is embarrassed and upset and does not really understand why her actions were a problem. She is also worried about her manual technique and concerned as to whether her technique will be good enough as she has not had very much practice.

Aesthetics	• Lucy wanted to get the allocated work done.
	• She was not fully aware of why her actions were problematic.
	• Lucy is as yet unaware of how important it is to take observations most thoroughly and accurately.
	• She is now feeling upset that her actions have caused a problem.
Personal	• Embarrassed, upset, uncertain feelings.
	• The desire to comply with mentor requests.
Ethics	• It seems very early in the process to have developed a value system.
	• Lucy is not fully aware of why taking manual observations is often so much more safe and accurate.
Empirics	• Sources of knowledge include manuals of clinical nursing procedures and Trust policy documents.
Reflexivity	• This situation is amplified by the vulnerability of Lucy's new position as guest within the placement.
	• With effective mentoring, Lucy could handle this better in similar situations in the future.
	• Lucy needs more practice with a manual sphygmomanometer and stethoscope.

The Davis model: a new experiential learning cycle

This is a new cyclical model (see Figure 9.3) with a slightly different cyclical structure from Gibbs' model (shown in Figure 9.2). It has an additional stage appraising the relevant evidence bases, which affirms the need for reflection to effect change.

This model shares some familiar features with the other reflective models we have considered. It starts with description and moves through a cyclical process towards considering opportunities for challenging or changing your practice in the future. We will now look at each one of these stages in some detail. The points made in each of these stages can also help you use and understand more fully the comparable stages in other models.

In order to reflect at a more critical level, you need to aim to work through all of the stages of your reflective model, as by doing so you will incrementally gather additional information to enhance your understanding of the experiences. This process can be worked through on your own, with your peers or mentors (or both).

Stage one: Describing the scenario

As we have already considered, the first stage of any reflective process will logically involve reviewing in detail the issue or scenario that you want to recall and can potentially learn from. This stage will be helped by the quality of your recall of events. Therefore, it is wise to write down the details as soon as you can, making the scenario anonymous where appropriate, as mandated by the NMC in order to protect confidentiality (NMC, 2008d). Stage one of the reflective learning cycle therefore involves documenting the story from practice, describing the sequence of events, charting the patient's journey through their pathway of care and/or describing a clinical situation you have encountered, describing in detail or highlighting the main points.

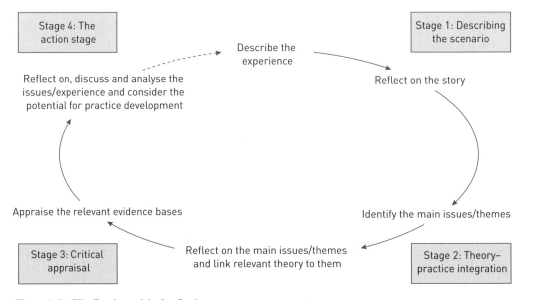

Figure 9.3: The Davis model of reflection

It is very important to accurately recall the story or issue that you want to reflect on. You might also reflect on why this particular issue is more memorable than any number of alternative scenarios. The more detail you put into stage one, the more fertile ground you will have on which to build your reflection. From that description you can then proceed to the next stage, considering main themes of interest and key words/phrases or issues, which can lead into a search for more information. The case study below shows an example of the firsts stage.

Case study: Yosef's first reflection on a clinical incident

In one of the high dependency units that I worked in I found that staff were entrenched in their routines, and sceptical of new evidence bases in favour of processing the workload as efficiently as possible. There was some very dominant staff working there, who had been there for a long time. I did not feel very welcome.

On one of the shifts a male patient, who was recovering from a myocardial infarction, went into cardiac arrest. The team on duty immediately went to his assistance. Ignoring the manual handling policy, the nurse in charge ordered the team of doctors and nurses on shift to 'haul' him from recliner chair to the bed for the purposes of starting cardiac resuscitation. I know this put all our backs at risk and we should slide him gently to the floor. But I was new to the unit and I said nothing. As we were lifting the dying man this same nurse shrieks in disgust, 'Why do these people let themselves get so fat!', referring to the patient. The resuscitation fails and the man dies.

Afterwards, I reflect as to whether this tirade may have been the last thing that the man heard as he was dying. I felt angry with this nurse at the time and still do resent her behaviour. I should have challenged her, but I didn't because I was a novice and felt vulnerable.

This is a really good example of a story that continues to trouble the conscience of this practitioner. Yosef is quite rightly angry and needs to defuse his anger. This may help him to transform this negative experience into a positive learning opportunity and transform future practice.

Stage two: Theory–practice integration

Stage two of the Davis model is concerned with making meaningful links between relevant theory and practice, looking at the similarities and differences between them and making sense of what has been found. This technical approach to reflection can be seen as embedded within other models, but here it is overtly cited because the evidence-based process is considered to be usefully implicit within its structure. At this stage you are going beyond description and starting to analyse why this particular event is prompting your memory sufficiently for you to want to write it down and learn from it. How does the practice that you have found in clinical areas compare or contrast with the theory that you may have already been taught or read about? Why are certain treatments that patients are receiving, or procedures, done in the ways in which you have observed or participated in? Are there persuasive evidence bases available to defend them? You could compare the local policies that govern practice within the clinical areas in which you have been working with national standards of care, looking at documents such as Department of Health reports. Have you found a difference? If so, what is the difference?

It may also be useful for you to search out additional current theory underpinning practice pertaining to your particular case studies, perhaps mapping these out into themes. You may want to search the literature (of published articles), looking particularly for best evidence of practice innovation in this area. This should give you plenty of additional information for discussion with your mentors and/or peers.

During this stage you can reflect on how theory and practice can complement and drive each other forward. Let's start to analyse the critical incident described above in stage one in the case study below.

Case study: Yosef's second reflection on a clinical incident

There are some clear themes that I could draw from the incident described in the case study above. This incident reveals issues with the attitude and behaviour of the senior nurse, which could be explored in terms of psychology, politics, morality and professionalism. Healthcare professionals are expected to display non-judgmental positive regard. There are also issues as to how much the patient may or may not have been aware of what was happening. If hearing is the last sense to leave us during cardiac arrest, then he might have heard himself being insulted just before he died. How can I find out if this is possible?

A literature search is the next obvious task that Yosef could logically undertake, online or in his local library. In Chapter 8 we find out what the literature search reveals. This includes engaging effectively with the first part of the evidence-based process – *searching for evidence* – as described in Chapter 8, p161.

Stage three: Critical appraisal

The Davis model explicitly includes a stage that is either implicit in or absent from other reflective models: that of critical appraisal. At this stage it is valuable to assess the quality of the evidence that you have found because you want your practice to be informed by effective evidence of good quality. This is a central part of working in an evidence-based way.

So how do you assess best evidence? Critical appraisal is a very important skill for nurses to develop, involving critical thinking. This, in turn, leads to deeper understanding. It involves the process of assessing and interpreting evidence, systematically considering the validity of the results and its relevance to your practice. You can consider how current theory and practice is supported by research and policy-making. Also consider issues such as clinical governance and evidence-based practice. How do you identify best practice? How do you establish that a source is a good piece of work and was based on good research and/or appropriate practice develop-ment? Is it appropriately timed? Does the practice need to change?

If you do not have any guidelines on critical appraisal skills, then it would be useful to find out more about these skills from books on research, some of which may be recommended to you by your tutors. These skills are also considered in Chapter 8 where you are introduced to a new set of critiquing frameworks.

Case study: Yosef's third reflection on a clinical incident

Yosef did find some relevant evidence that helped him to deconstruct what was happening in the scenario. While appraising the evidence, he was able to reflect at a much deeper level on how this critical appraisal stage influenced his opinions of the evidence so far gathered. He thereafter felt better able to evaluate how this developed his feelings about the practice he had observed within the case study. So there was much to gain from engaging with the second part of the evidence-based process: appraising sources of evidence *– as described in Chapter 8, pages 162–3.*

Stage four: The action stage

Stage four of the Davis model is consistent with the logical last stage of any reflective model, which invites you to consider whether action needs to be taken to challenge and change practice. This may involve considering how practice can change and develop in the light of fresh evidence. At this stage, think about and reflect on how you can support best practice. This practice development stage may be something that you feel you can only think about in theory and discuss with your peers as potential for action. However, as you continue through your pre-registration studies, progress through more placements and see your confidence grow, you may feel more able to discuss practice development opportunities with your mentors. They may be very happy to listen to your ideas and suggestions. At this stage, you could reflect on how this process may support or change practice, for yourself and potentially within the clinical area.

Case study: Yosef's fourth reflection on a clinical incident

Yosef now feels much better informed and prepared for the future with this new information. He feels he is in a better position to challenge such poor practice in future. Nevertheless, he is cautious because he knows that change may be difficult to effect quickly. He starts to consider how junior staff can legitimately, but also safely, challenge senior staff, when they fail to perform as effective role models.

Activity 9.4   *Reflection*

Having now gone through all four stages of the new reflective learning cycle, have your opinions of what you have found in the clinical incident changed? If so, in what ways? What do you think Yosef would do if he encountered a similar situation in the future?

An outline answer is provided at the end of the chapter.

One place to start when challenging the clinical incident described in stage one would be to consider the impact on staff development of improving interpersonal skills, which might impact on the senior nurse's attitude. Perhaps this is a staff training issue? Alternatively, her actions could be considered a breach of professional conduct and the suggestion could be made that the senior nurse should have been reported for misconduct to her manager and potentially also the NMC. Since she was in breach of the duty of care by not acting in the best interests of the patient or co-operating with her colleagues, the case might well be followed up. This could also be considered to be a resource issue: should patients be in soft reclining chairs in a clinical area from which they cannot be moved easily? Considering the many themes we raised at stage two, it is clear that following up on these themes will influence the direction of the recommendations that might be suggested.

The rationale for the cycle

To close the loop on this cycle, you would now have three choices as represented after stage four in Figure 9.3.

1. If the process was successful, then the practice development, either individually for you or collectively within the clinical area, is taken forward and the learning loop closes.
2. If the process was useful but was not completed or not satisfactorily concluded, the cycle can be repeated. More information may be needed or come to light, so the cycle may need to be repeated.
3. If the process did not meet your learning needs, an alternative model and/or approach may be necessary. You might prefer to use Driscoll's model, which is straightforward and highly effective, or like the personal and emotive emphasis in Gibbs' model or the diverse detail of Johns' model.

Writing and recording your reflections

You should keep some written examples of reflective practice and other critically developmental activities, compiled over time and kept as evidence of ongoing progress. The maintenance of a portfolio of evidence that includes written reflective accounts is part of the requirement for you to demonstrate full engagement with lifelong learning (NMC, 2008d). The next chapter will therefore consider how to provide further evidence of your development and suggest good practice regarding how to record reflection and other activities within a portfolio of evidence.

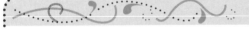

Chapter summary

We started this chapter by considering the nature and purpose of reflection, acknowledging that reflection is a mandatory expectation within professional practice and aligned with the requirement within Domain 4: to maintain knowledge, develop skills and engage with lifelong learning. The focus of this has been on understanding how to learn effectively from experience, where appropriate, and recording this by reflecting on action. This can form the basis of a learning log cataloguing theory and practice. Reflection can facilitate opportunities to bring theory and practice together; to see how they can link up and challenge each other, working towards delivering evidence-based care.

continued opposite . . .

continued . . . ●●

Within this chapter we have considered several models that are all designed to guide and structure reflection. This résumé of three of the most widely cited available models, culminated in reviewing a newer model defined by a simple four-stage process. Reflective models usually commence with description, which invites retrospective consideration of stories of, from and within practice. Arguably, any reflection should move beyond description of the event, through a dynamic and iterative cycle or process; which only completes upon consideration of the capacity for change. Engaging with practice development is not easy. It will involve consideration of the original practice, evaluation of attitudes to changing this practice, personal evaluation of the new practice and the rationale for the change. All of these processes can be challenging. So strategies to enhance reflection include using a reflective model to structure this self-inquiry, summarising relevant theory and practice, developing critical reading skills, including paraphrasing and appraising relevant supporting evidence. Access to evidence bases, information literacy and familiarity with the process of practice development will also support the reflection.

Activities: Brief outline answers

Activity 9.2 (pages 177–8)

Some possible explanations for the use of jargon in handover include:

* time pressure to get large amounts of clinical information conveyed within the handover – a great deal of information can be shared within these inter-shift communications, so there may be some justification of handovers in terms of potential time-saving;
* power: the use of jargon is exclusive and marginalising;
* established routine that becomes entrenched and unquestioned;
* aspirations to portray nursing as more scientific.

Grace could ask her mentor, Staff Nurse Kaur, for an orientation pack to help her feel more comfortable prior to future handovers. This would help to structure her self-study and make her feel better informed and prepared for the next shift. Grace can then use this learning to turn a potential negative experience towards a positive outcome.

Activity 9.3 (page 183)

Jo-Yan might have to consider approaching her personal tutor at the university to discuss the possibility of further practice within the clinical skills lab or accessing counselling and/or desensitisation techniques. There are some fields of nursing in which giving injections is a rare event, but it is still a skill that Jo-Yan needs to learn and be assessed on. Her mentor may turn out to an expert source of support and help Jo-Yan to practise injection technique, while being carefully supervised.

Activity 9.4 (page 189)

Your responses might have taken you to biological, psychological or sociological theory. You might have considered whether hearing is the last sense to go and, if so, how we know that. You might have looked at the way that nursing teams work in practice and how positions of power can be abused, particularly by experienced but work-weary practitioners who have become spiritually or emotionally disconnected from their work. Whether you looked at ethics, attitudes or standards of conduct, hopefully this story initiated a great deal of internal or group dialogue. Yosef may very well have to make a difficult decision now: whether to report the incident to the unit manager or contact the NMC for advice. He would be well advised to also contact his personal tutor at the university and the placement support unit.

Further reading

Driscoll, J (2007) Chapter 2: Supported reflective learning: the essence of clinical supervision?, in Driscoll, JJ (ed.) *Practising Clinical Supervision: A reflective approach for healthcare professionals* (2nd edition), pp27–52. Edinburgh: Baillière Tindall, Elsevier.

An important resource that offers current thinking on reflection related to clinical supervision.

Driscoll, J and Teh, B (2001) The potential of reflective practice to develop individual orthopaedic nurse practitioners and their practice. *Journal of Orthopaedic Nursing*, 5: 95–103.

Driscoll's model is discussed in more depth within this short article.

Howatson-Jones, L (2010) *Reflective Practice in Nursing*. Exeter: Learning Matters.

Another book in the same series as this book (Transforming Nursing Practice), which looks at reflective practice in more detail. A great introduction to the subject, short and easy to read.

Johns, C (2004) *Becoming a Reflective Practitoner* (2nd edition). Oxford: Blackwell.

Chris Johns discusses the nature of reflective practice and his model.

Johns, C (2006) *Engaging Reflection in Practice*. Oxford: Blackwell.

This is the further development of Johns' theories on reflection and discusses reflective models.

Taylor, BJ (2006) *Reflective Practice: A guide for nurses and midwives* (2nd edition). Berkshire: Open University Press.

This book is a really reader-friendly and well-supported text, written by an acknowledged expert within this subject area. While the book is quite short, it is full of recognition of the growing evidence bases supporting the value of reflective practice.

Useful websites

http://hsc.uwe.ac.uk/net/mentor/Default.aspx?pageid=117

Includes some useful information on reflective models, including simple diagrams.

www.supervisionandcoaching.com/

The site of John Driscoll Consulting and a free resource for all nurses and those involved in supporting reflective practice and professional supervision in healthcare.

Chapter 10

Portfolios and personal development plans: keeping track of your learning

Nicola Davis

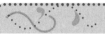

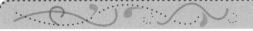

NMC Essential Skills Clusters

This chapter will address the following ESC:

Cluster: Care, compassion and communication

1. As partners in the care process, people can trust the newly registered nurse to provide collaborative care based on the highest standards, knowledge and competence.

By the first progression point:

1. Articulates the underpinning values of *The Code: Standards of conduct, performance and ethics for nurses and midwives (the code)* (NMC, 2008b).
2. Works within limitations of the role and recognises own level of competence.
3. Promotes a professional image.
4. Shows respect for others.

By the second progression point:

7. Uses professional support structures to learn from experience and make appropriate adjustments.
5. People can trust the newly registered graduate nurse to engage with them in a warm, sensitive and compassionate way.

By entry to the register

13. Through reflection and evaluation demonstrates commitment to personal and professional development and lifelong learning.

Chapter aims

By the end of this chapter, you should be able to:

• demonstrate a fundamental understanding of the purpose and content of portfolios and personal development plans;
• recognise the importance of lifelong learning in career and personal development;
• understand why portfolio development is important in practice development;
• start compiling a portfolio of learning achievement.

Introduction

Scenario

Imagine that you are already in your first staff nurse post. It is twelve months since qualifying and you feel that it is time to move on to a new post to gain more diverse experience. The first year after qualifying can be very busy and anxiety provoking, with so much to learn. There has not been time to keep your portfolio up to date. However, it is risky going to interviews without a current portfolio. Now, as quickly as possible, you are going to have to catch up with collecting evidence of your development over the last year.

Nurses, like all healthcare professionals, are expected to engage in learning and development throughout their career. As a nurse you will be responsible for developing your practice in order to keep up to date with changes in theory and in practice, as an ongoing process that is known as lifelong learning. Lifelong learning involves independent inquiry, internal challenge, expanding knowledge and developing understanding, skills and competency. This involves maintaining a long-term interest in advancing your practice. The NMC (2008b) requires that all nurses maintain an active interest in advancing their own learning and development in order to develop their scope of practice. Portfolios can provide a forum in which such development can be recorded. In addition to this, all registered nurses should contribute towards creating an environment in which learning can flourish. A commitment to recording this learning will contribute to this responsibility by role modelling.

Nursing students are also expected to start engaging in portfolio development right from the beginning of their studies, taking responsibility for forging ahead with their own development (NMC, 2008b, 2008c). Full engagement with lifelong learning will demonstrate your commitment to delivering quality care and therefore acting in the best interests of your patients or clients. Completing a portfolio during the pre-registration period of study is good practice. In order to fulfil NMC requirements post-registration, it is mandatory for all qualified nurses to maintain both a personal and professional portfolio, which could be audited by the NMC at any time. You need to be fully prepared for this. Within this portfolio you should include clear evidence of both active and experiential learning, including structured, written reflective accounts. In this chapter, we will consider why this process is necessary and how compiling a portfolio can incorporate a personal development plan that drives your development.

What is a portfolio?

A portfolio is a collection of evidence that demonstrates your professional development. Over time, the portfolio can become a very large document, so it will need a good index. There can be two broad sections to the portfolio: the personal and the professional. Both of these sections should be of equal value to you, but they will be developed for very different reasons.

The personal portfolio

The personal portfolio is essentially a private document, which includes individual records of the development of your skills, knowledge, attitudes, understanding and achievements. It may also be the best location to store your structured written accounts of individual case studies and critical incident reviews. The portfolio is an ideal place for evidence of your written reflective accounts.

Alongside tangible evidence of reflective practice, other critically developmental activities compiled over time can be kept safe and secure within the portfolio, contributing evidence of ongoing progress.

You might want to consider compiling your own learning contract with yourself. Consider what you need to achieve, assess what the priorities are and plan a timescale for achievement, bearing in mind the associated resource implications. Also consider what type of learner you are. This may include thinking about where you learn best and what type of learning opportunities have suited you best among those you have experienced thus far.

Activity 10.1 *Reflection*

Think about something that you have had to learn that you found very challenging to complete – for example, learning to drive or a new outdoor activity such as rock climbing. At the beginning of the process you might have felt quite daunted by the challenge. Make some notes on how you overcame that initial anxiety.

As this is based on your own reflection, there is no outline answer provided.

The professional portfolio

The 'professional profile' part of the portfolio is a public document and you need to design it with this in mind. You will need to select evidence that is structured in such a way that the document can be shared with a specific audience, so it needs to be succinct, clear and presented to a high standard. It may include, for example:

- accounts of professional experience and direct observations of practice development;
- shared ideas and opinions that have been discussed with colleagues;
- evaluations of new working methods, which may be currently being trialled within your clinical area.

However, the way it will really serve you well in the future is in that it documents specific achievements in your qualifications, clinical skills profiles and key transferable skills. From this evidence, a potential employer can assess your contribution to nursing and what you have to offer them. You will therefore want to maintain a portfolio of evidence that includes written reflection, which forms part of demonstrating full engagement with your development through lifelong learning (NMC, 2008c). We will therefore now consider why you need to clearly demonstrate your development and record all of your progress within a portfolio of evidence.

Why you need to compile a portfolio

At regular intervals throughout your career, you will have to challenge yourself and consider whether you could improve your practice. Your knowledge will need to evolve as demands upon your practice change and you have to learn more in order to develop. It is an expectation of professional practice that you can defend your practice and so you truly need to develop your understanding of what informs this. The process of lifelong learning will expand your skills, and in doing so make you a more competent nurse.

Portfolio development is a very important way of demonstrating your personal commitment to your own professional development and to the process of lifelong learning. It conveys an impression of your personal investment in professional practice and an active interest in maintaining an accurate record of your lifelong learning. Therefore, it is a requirement of professional nursing practice (NMC, 2008c), which requires engagement with the delivery of current and credible quality care. Maintaining a portfolio is also useful for your future career planning, for marketing yourself for potential career options. The way that you present yourself in your public portfolio is as a glimpse of the type of professional you are, so you want to show you take care and pay attention. The portfolio can demonstrate the ongoing development of your clinical and key transferable skills, which you may later present at interviews. It will help you prepare for individual performance reviews such as annual reviews and appraisals. Therefore, your portfolio should clearly and carefully document the progression of your career. During your nursing studies, your university may also require you to keep a portfolio or a personal development plan to track your progress. This may include an ongoing record of achievement, which is used as part of the assessment of your practice and achievement of the outcomes for each part of the programme. It is an NMC mandatory requirement for all nursing programme providers to keep an ongoing record of achievement for each student (NMC, 2010). Both the portfolio and ongoing record of achievement can be used to track your learning progress in a formal and informal way.

In Chapter 8 we considered how healthcare professionals need to be able to defend their practice. This means that decision-making needs to be transparent and that there needs to be clear rationales for taking certain courses of action. This type of developmental work can be documented and help to build up a profile that really shows the advances you are making in your development.

Seven good reasons to compile a portfolio

1   To demonstrate clear compliance with NMC requirements, both within your nursing programme and when you qualify.
2   To help plan your career from the very beginning and throughout.
3   To contribute to your appraisals as they occur regularly throughout your career.
4   To market yourself for future employment and development opportunities.
5   To develop your scope of practice, and evidence for that progression.
6   To keep your knowledge up to date.
7   Personal development: taking pride in your achievements.

Table 10.1: Seven good reasons to compile a portfolio

Case study

Staff Nurse Judy has been working permanent nights for the past year. She quietly reviews her current skills profiles and appreciates that she has been refining her ability to administer medications, complete advanced procedures such as male catheterisation and manage the shift. However, when Judy is asked to mentor a student who has asked to do extra night shifts, Judy realises upon reviewing the student's assessment documents that there are several areas of practice that she herself has not been practising regularly and this worries her. Judy supports the student for the next couple of weeks but then asks the Ward Manager if she can do some reorientation day shifts soon in order to refresh her skills.

Past, present and future

From the case study above, it should be clear that no practitioner can 'rest easy' imagining that their skills profiles will remain current, unless they take active steps to make that happen. You may be aware of your legal responsibility to document the care you give as evidence that the care was given. The portfolio is an equally important tool to protect you and your career. A personal development plan does not only look back to the past, but turns the focus away from what you have achieved towards considering, with specific goals, what you can do in order to develop yourself in the future. Therefore, within this plan you can set in place realistic milestones for achievement over time. Later in this chapter, specific features of such a plan will be considered, particularly with regard to the types of competency profiles that it may include. When setting goals for specific learning objectives, you need to set realistic timescales and also think about the necessary resources, be they time, money or childcare. Such specific and careful planning will help to focus you on exactly what you want to achieve and how.

Why is a portfolio so important?

A portfolio is important for you politically, professionally, clinically and ethically.

We have already discussed why you need to carefully and accurately track your progress towards becoming a professional nurse in terms of helping you to prepare for a future of professional accountable practice. Keeping a portfolio should ensure that the evidence is kept together within a well-presented folder, which is logistically sensible. We have already considered how pre-sentation matters because if the portfolio is well presented, it conveys an impression of due care and attention. Being careful is an important attribute for any professional, but what may also underpin the value of this portfolio is that the record should be complete and kept readily accessible.

The political perspective

You are expected to be part of a process that enables clinical governance to be an overt reality. Both the Department of Health and the NMC expect a commitment to EBP to form a central pillar of that. You can record your development in your portfolio and thereby demonstrate that you are challenging yourself to change, be proactive and deliver quality care. This will help you present yourself as a fully accountable practitioner who can defend your practice if challenged.

The professional perspective

Providing evidence for your development is good for you professionally because this is part of a process that verifies what you have to offer to nursing, an important consideration for anyone who may assess or employ you in the future. For example, you will need to take a representative extract of your portfolio when you are interviewed for any job related to nursing. So this process can be justified professionally in terms of potential career advancement. You are moving from a position of responsibility towards accountability once registered, so getting into the good habit of timely and effective documentation of your achievements should become embedded within your practice. This position of substantial responsibility requires a high level of professionalism. A well-compiled and presented portfolio will show that you are well organised and committed to the delivery of high quality care. This agreement with the expectations of professional practice, including 'going the extra mile' and documenting progress, is important in affirming the claim that nursing has to be considered a profession. So this can be seen to have a political advantage.

The clinical and ethical perspectives

A well-structured portfolio is also good for you clinically because it catalogues your individual commitment to being effective in delivering high quality care. We have already considered how an integral part of that incorporates a commitment to pursuing evidence-based care, an important part of keeping you and your practice current. This demonstrates an ongoing commitment to contributing to delivering quality of care, which is overtly in the best interests of the client and is ethically defensible. The NMC expects nurses to act in the best interests of clients, in a manner that involves fundamentally aiming to do good and preventing harm. As we discussed earlier in Chapter 8, the stages of EBP should help you to identify and deliver quality care, through finding evidence, appraising evidence and reflecting on how applicable that evidence is. All of those stages are equally important, all effected by developing specific skills and all of which can be recorded within your portfolio. One of your most important starting points might be the ongoing record of learning achievement you complete through your clinical placements. This set of documents may explicitly state what you need to achieve and you will need to provide evidence for each achievement, citing current relevant literature to support your assertions as to what constitutes best practice.

Activity 10.2   *Decision-making*

Julian is a first-year nursing student who is at the beginning of his second practice learning opportunity. He has achieved most of his year one learning outcomes within the first practice learning opportunity and is now looking forward to making further progress within this placement. However, his current mentor wants to see him demonstrate all of those skills again.

Is this defensible in terms of demonstrating maintenance of learning, or is it unnecessary duplication of effort for both mentor and mentee?

In what ways could Julian's portfolio of learning achievement help him in this situation?

An outline answer is provided at the end of the chapter.

We will return to some of the issues raised in Activity 10.2 later in the chapter, but for now will turn to considering what to include in a good contents list for a portfolio.

The contents of the portfolio

We have already established that this complex document will need a good index. It also needs to be updated regularly. The contents list should help your reader navigate through the parts of the document that you are happy to share. So while you are devising a clear and accurate contents list, consider how you will manage the distinct sections your future readers can select from.

Your portfolio should be divided up clearly and logically. It should be kept within a cover or file in order to maintain the quality of the contents effectively. We have already considered how much presentation matters and that it contributes to the impression you convey. Therefore, try to think of ways to make your portfolio eye-catching and succinct yet also informative, aiming to keep the reader interested and focused on the quality of your work.

As there are conventionally two main sections of the portfolio (personal and professional), you might want to present these two very different sections in different ways. You could use two files, with the professional section backed up by electronic records. You need to think particularly carefully about how to store and present the professional section, which will be shared with other people for a variety of reasons. The personal section, which can be 'closed' or private, could quite legitimately be in one hard copy form, to which only you have access. How much of the personal portfolio you share is up to you, but bear in mind that there are some parts of your personal learning journey that either cannot or should not be shared because they are so very personal to you. All parts of your portfolio should be made suitably anonymous in terms of place and person. This is vital to ensure confidentiality. To do otherwise could be a risk if it should come to light that sensitive information is disclosed within your personal records.

Both of these sections are equally valuable to you as they contribute to your development and can inform your understanding of yourself as the 'developing professional'. Let's look at a possible overview of potential contents list for both main sections.

The personal profile

Table 10.2 offers a possible contents list for your personal profile section.

Contents of a Personal Profile
Self-awareness raising activities, such as strengths, needs, opportunities and barriers to learning (SNOB) analysis
Evidence of development of knowledge and understanding, attitudes and skills (including key transferable skills), conducive to professional practice
Achievement of specific personal goals, e.g. information literacy
Critical incident analysis and case study reviews from personal practice
Personal analysis and evaluation of significant learning events
Learning styles analysis

Table 10.2: Possible contents list for a personal profile

This personal section may include individual records of the development of practical skills, knowledge, attitudes, understanding and achievements. From these records you might select those that you are happy to share in your public profile. The personal profile is the correct place to collate accounts of activities that have helped you to better understand yourself as a person, learner and nursing student. It is appropriate that you contemplate where, when and how you learn best, consider what type of team worker you are and consider the barriers and enablers to your learning. This may well help you to capitalise on the opportunities with which you are faced. Consider the following scenario.

Scenario

Matilda is a mature student who has decided to train to be a nurse now that her three children have all started school. She can get to the university campus for 9.30 a.m. after dropping the children at school, and her mother will help look after the children out of school hours when she is on placements. She still cleans her own house and does all of the shopping because her partner is in full-time work and comes home very tired every evening. When Matilda is home in the evening she cooks the tea, baths the children and reads them their bedtime stories. By the time she has finished it is usually after 9 p.m. and she has already been busy for over twelve hours and is too tired to study. The TV is on in the lounge and the whole house seems too noisy to concentrate. If this situation does not ease she is worried about how she will get her essays written. Matilda is worried about what she can do.

Where is Matilda going to study? In Chapter 7 we looked at the many and varied services the library offers. Matilda might find that independent study in the private study areas at her university library or the district library close to where she lives really pays off. Alternatively, she could arrange for one of her family to take the children out on Saturday afternoons to give her some additional study time. Ultimately, her partner may have to find the reserves to help more around the house as well.

It is important that your personal profile should include structured written reflective accounts of individual case studies and critical incident reviews. These reflections should analyse and evaluate scenarios that you have encountered in practice. As discussed in Chapters 8 and 9, keeping such records will help you capitalise fully on your practical experiences, helping you to learn more from them. As these are private contributions to the portfolio and deeply personal, you may not ever want or need to share them with anyone else. However, it would still be wise to maintain anonymity of place and person.

The personal profile may include personal accounts of direct observations of others' practice, including ideas about how nursing practice might be better in the future and any opinions you are forming. You may also want to include evaluations of new working methods that you have read about within current, credible sources of literature, while you are forming an opinion about whether they might work in areas of practice that you have directly encountered.

In your personal portfolio you can afford to be honest with yourself about your strengths and future learning needs. You might also want to compile a learning diary of your experiences during your studies, which could culminate in a fascinating chronicle of the time building up towards your career. It is very important to see the process of developing the personal portfolio as both empowering and positive for your development, even though some of those activities might reveal gaps in your knowledge and skills. The reflective accounts in the personal part of your portfolio need not be exclusively focused on issues of concern and may well represent a more balanced evaluation of your individual abilities and potential to offer effective care. You can and should reflect on positive developments as well – for example, appreciation of successful development to date, and evaluations of attitude changes you may have noticed. Within healthcare practice you will experience many clinical scenarios from which you can learn. Sometimes that reflective learning will be very personal and you may benefit from thinking about it alone and privately.

As you develop you may consider what your current abilities are and how you can build on those strengths in future. You might find this an even more illuminating process when you consider your level of self-awareness. A tool to help you with this is called the Johari Window (Luft and Ingham, 1955). This tool is designed to enhance self-awareness of interpersonal skills and relationships, and can increase your understanding of how you communicate and interact with other people, leading you to 'describe' your personality. The tool facilitates reflection on how much of ourselves we are conscious of and also how much others might see in us, which we may or may not be conscious of. As such, it may form a valuable part of our self-development.

This tool reminds us that other people may perceive us in very different ways from those in which we view ourselves. If you would like to know more about this tool, then go to **www.business balls.com/johariwindowmodel.htm**.

You can use the section of your portfolio where you keep your written reflections to explore how you are changing as a person as you progress through your studies. You may be happy to share your awareness of your strengths, but considering your learning needs and development opportunities might be something that you want to consider initially on your own. You then have the option of considering when and from whom you need to seek help and advice.

1. Open/free area	2. Blind area
3. Hidden area	4 Unknown area

Figure 10.1: The Johari Window model

Activity 10.3 — *Reflection*

Try to imagine how other people perceive you. Do you convey the impression that you think you do? Try this activity with a peer with whom you feel comfortable. Write down what you think your style of communication is and then what your partner's style of communication is. Exchange notes. Do they match?

As this is a personal activity, there is no outline answer provided.

The public profile

The outward-facing part of the portfolio, or 'public profile', is a public document and therefore you will need to construct it with a potential audience in mind. This is important for all the reasons we have already discussed – for example, you need to be prepared to take it into interviews and appraisals. Once you become registered, the NMC can request to review your professional portfolio as evidence that you are meeting the requirements of continuing professional development (CPD) standards required to maintain registration as a nurse.

Concept summary: why sharing portfolios is important

- **Professional regulation**: the NMC expects you to give evidence for your lifelong learning and development, and this usually starts during your pre-registration studies. The NMC can request to see your portfolio pre- or post-registration.
- **Career progression**: maintaining a portfolio will help to better demonstrate your achievements in an accessible manner.
- **Educational assessment**: to demonstrate an overview of the progress of your learning as part of the formal assessment process – portfolios can be submitted as components of assessment on some modules.
- **Accountability**: once registered you can be held accountable for the quality of care that you deliver and your portfolio can be called as evidence if your competency is challenged via professional or legal proceedings.

The following example will help to illustrate how the professional portfolio can help you as a registered nurse in terms of future employability.

Activity 10.4   *Critical thinking*

Staff Nurse Francine Bauby has decided to apply for a new nursing position in the Rapid Response Community Nursing Team because she has worked on her current ward for three years and would like to experience a new area of nursing practice. She wants to make a good impression at the interview and is aware that a 30-minute interview (which is what she has been told to expect) is not very long in which to prove your worth as a potential employee. Francine looks back over her current portfolio. It contains her certificate confirming nurse training, staff development attendance certificates, two completed self-assessment packs from a nursing journal and some photocopied articles.

What could Francine do to improve it?

An outline answer is provided at the end of the chapter.

We have considered how portfolio development is a very important way of demonstrating ongoing professional development, conveying evidence of advancing professional practice and maintaining a record of lifelong learning. It is also an important way to prepare for individual performance reviews such as annual appraisals. You may find that you are expected to meet annually with your personal tutor during your studies, in order to review your progress within theory and practice modules. Now you know that the portfolio is useful for career planning, for marketing yourself in the future for potential career options and evidencing the ongoing development of your core and transferable skills, it is important now to consider what your public profile might contain.

Content and presentation of the public profile

As the portfolio is a resource to be used for several different reasons it should be divided up clearly and logically. You might like to design it as quite a large collection from which you can draw bespoke section copies for various purposes. Try to think of ways to make these sections of the portfolio eye-catching and informative, aiming to keep the reader interested and focused on your work.

When you are going to performance reviews, appraisals or interviews, you might consider having a smaller, removable and therefore portable profile from the portfolio. You could take a copy of this to the interview as you then might feel comfortable to leave it with your interviewers. This shows both pride in your achievements and consideration for the interviewers' finite time to conduct the interview. After the interview, leaving a profile with them will remind them of how organised you are, with the bonus that you respect how busy they are too. We have already stressed the importance of the public profile being structured with due consideration of sharing this document with specific audiences. Let us now consider in more detail the possible contents of this part of your portfolio. Table 10.3 lists the contents of a typical public profile section. This is a suggested order for items in a portfolio, but so long as you provide a contents page you can order the items as you wish.

We will look now look at each of these contents in a little more detail.

Curriculum vitae (CV)

This should be a 'snapshot' of your achievements, including qualifications, personal strengths, working interests and competencies. Your CV should be succinct and eye-catching, operating as an efficient overview of your best features. It should have your contact details at the top. It is your best chance of getting someone's attention quickly and you should use it to focus constructively and realistically on your strengths. You can include some general information. For example, you might say that you possess a full clean driving licence as this says something about you – it indicates that you can not only drive but do so safely. This is a personal quality worth having that gives more insight into you as a person than you might realise. See Figure 10.2 for an example of the front page of a CV.

Evidence of formal accredited learning

When you study for credit-bearing courses and modules you should receive written confirmation and/or certificates to verify that achievement. Such evidence should be kept with care and be well presented. The professional portfolio is a good place to keep it, although you do need

Contents of a Public Profile

Curriculum vitae

Ideally, a succinct one-page presentation summarising your knowledge and skills, located at the front of the portfolio. This is your initial sales pitch and first opportunity to make a good impression. There are a variety of standard templates available to help you construct a CV or you could consider having it professionally produced, which would clearly have cost implications.

Evidence of formal accredited learning, including certificates

This demonstrates your progress through formal education and the development of propositional knowledge. It should verify your claim to specific qualifications.

Evidence of informal learning

This includes notes from seminars and presentations, which can often be very important in encouraging self-study and self-assessment of your learning. This should not include hand-outs of lecture notes because you would not have produced them yourself.

A reflective learning journal

This would be compiled over time to track your progress through some specific learning opportunities. It guards against forgetting important learning that has taken place and avoids hindsight bias. It might include a learning diary kept during group learning activities, which you are happy to share because it demonstrates your collaborative abilities and teamworking skills.

Evidence of all of the key transferable skills

These skills are particularly literacy, communication, information technology and information literacy. This book has taken the opportunity to consider all of these skills in order to highlight their importance to you in enhancing your ability to nurse well.

Critical appraisals of current, credible relevant sources of evidence

This shows the means of moving towards understanding and constructive evaluations of new ways of working.

Written reflective accounts, including critical incident analysis

These show the capacity to learn in depth from experience. They would need to be made anonymous to protect all individuals involved.

Presentation, and progression, of specific clinical learning and skills development

These build a competency profile, which shows increasing evidence of your employability. Your ongoing record of clinical learning in placements should form the backbone of this.

Table 10.3: Contents of a typical public profile section of the portfolio

Figure 10.2: Front page of a CV

> **CURRICULUM VITAE**
>
> **Lilley Snowflake**
> **7 Caviary Avenue**
> **Little Lane**
> **Hawton on the Hill**
> **BS123 4BC**
>
> A highly organised and enthusiatic nurse, with excellent interpersonal and information technology skills.
>
> **Qualifications**
> Registered Nurse (Adult), Cherry Orchard College, 09/2005
> BSc (Hons) Nursing Studies, University of the Western Highlands, 07/ 2007
> Teaching & Assessing (Level M module), 04/2008
>
> **Experience**
> Staff Nurse, General Surgical Ward, 09/2005–03/2009
> Staff Nurse, Rapid Response Team, 03/2009–present
> Member of the Royal College of Nursing
>
> **Personal**
> Full clean driving licence
> Voluntary worker at Hawthorns Homeless Shelter

photocopies as well. If you get into the habit of maintaining such records in one safe place, there is less chance you will lose them. As you progress through your studies, the safe compilation of such records will become increasingly important. A potential future employer will be impressed that you are able to keep good records over time.

Evidence of informal learning

This is an extremely important consideration. As active working adults, we are surrounded by learning opportunities all the time, but with information overload you could lose vast quantities of these learning opportunities by not recording them and therefore learning from them. When considering challenges in practice, you may identify workload stressors, educational needs and barriers to development that are of concern to you, and as a result you feel motivated to work on. These may be worthy of either individual or group practice development.

There are several exercises that you can do within this section of the portfolio. You could consider your present strengths and how you plan to challenge them by carrying out a SNOB analysis of strengths, needs, opportunities and barriers, as seen in Figure 10.3.

Make notes under each heading. You could consider your style of learning and whether your experiences within current studies challenge or inhibits that. We mentioned the Johari Window earlier and if you do a search online for self-assessment tools, you will find many other freely available materials to try. See the Useful websites section at the end of this chapter for a good example of a website offering a variety of self-assessment materials.

Strengths	Needs
Opportunities	Barriers

Figure 10.3: Template for an assessment of strengths, needs, opportunities and barriers

Learning journal

This might be a very personal diary in your portfolio, and you may decide to keep it private. However, you might also take it to group learning situations such as enquiry, problem or work-based learning. You could view this as a key opportunity to maintain a record of the emotional impact of working within healthcare, considering your thoughts and feelings.

Evidence of key transferable skills

This part of your portfolio should be well presented, professionally maintained and displayed. In being well written it will provide evidence of your literacy. Communicating well on paper demonstrates a further strand to your interpersonal skills development. If the profile is word-processed, then this shows further evidence of your IT skills. In being well evidenced, including only those items that you have worked on personally, the portfolio will show your capacity to engage proactively with providing clear rationales for action. Developing your portfolio will also help you to practise many of the important skills that need to be maintained for assessments in theory and practice throughout your studies. During annual reviews with your personal tutor, you should bring in your portfolio to demonstrate this, just as you will in annual appraisals once you are registered with the NMC.

Appraisals of evidence and evaluations of new ways of working

The process of critical appraisal is discussed at length in Chapter 8. Within your portfolio you can provide evidence of your ability to engage with all three main stages of the evidence-based practice process. Your information literacy skills, discussed above, help you to initiate a satisfactory 'find' when searching for evidence. Your critical appraisal skills help you to analyse and evaluate the quality of these sources once you have found them. Amid information overload, the all-important quality assurance process is vital. Evidencing this within your portfolio demonstrates your commitment to delivering evidence-based care in the best interests of the patient. You need to show you are willing to move forward as nursing knowledge and technology progresses.

Written reflective accounts, and critical incident analysis

As discussed in Chapter 8, written accounts of your reflections demonstrate your capacity to record events accurately, identify the important themes from which to learn and explore further and consider whether or how you might see certain practices improve. This is vital in developing into a well-rounded reflective professional who contemplates change when it is necessary.

Competency profile

This should set out clear, articulate statements of specific learning outcomes related to each and every skill that you need to learn and demonstrate (see example in Table 10.4 below). These should be clear both to you and those who assess your ability to master the competencies, particularly with practice. In reality, during your studies this may be provided by your course leaders. It is good practice to display your achievement in specific competencies in this way, and it is reassuring to you and others that you are only delivering practices that you know are safe and identifying areas that need more attention and development. Once you are qualified you may have to work through a similar set of competencies, during a period of preceptorship. This may well form part of what can be termed a personal development plan or PDP.

The personal development plan (PDP)

The PDP is a future-facing section of a portfolio. It considers what needs to be achieved to accord with the specific expectations of a role. As discussed above, it should include specific competency statements. These can be assessed by a mentor and/or assessor. It is important to see the PDP as

Specific competency	Assessment date	Assessor signature	Review date
Able to safely engage in sole administration of medication			
Understands Trust policy on administration of medication			
Understands Trust policy on near-miss and drug error reporting			
Understands common routes of medication administration and associated techniques			
Understands Trust controlled drug policy			
Understands Trust policy on management of anaphylaxis			
Maintains working knowledge of basic pharmacology			

Table 10.4: Illustration of competency statements: medicines management

a mechanism not only to motivate and record your progress but also to protect all key stakeholders. You need to be safe and well supervised within practice, and to act in the best interests of the patient or client. The PDP should help you to make that happen because it should have specific goals embedded within it.

So right from the very beginning of your studies you need to get into the good habit of documenting your learning in the same way that you will be taught to achieve and maintain high quality records when you document the care you deliver. You can view this portfolio as a storehouse of evidence to impress both yourself and those who will assess you during and after your studies. It may also help to demonstrate progress and avoid you having to backtrack in practice, reproving your abilities. In Activity 10.2, we considered the plight of Julian, who faced this very issue. If he has kept a good portfolio so far, his new mentor might be reassured that he already has some skills and progress to help him achieve new skills.

How can you make this happen?

Having considered all the features of portfolio and PDP building, what features in yourself can you develop to help create this resource? You need to be able to honestly and constructively self-evaluate your progress. An example of this might be considering your current level of inter-personal skills, including assertiveness skills, and assessing where the development opportunities might be. You will need to believe in yourself and have the confidence to prioritise your learning and development; within the portfolio you can demonstrate your ability to articulate your development and objectives. If we relate this to Activity 10.4 (page 203), this could lead Staff Nurse Bauby to explore the nature and necessity of self-appraisal and appreciate her developing expertise within nursing practice. By progressing through this rigorous self-evaluation, you should be actively and meaningfully learning from experience by contemplating what is happening in the here and now and considering how this can be challenged in the future – the essence of critical reflection. In Chapter 9, we considered how important critical reflection was to the achievement of double loop learning and the development of self. Double-loop learning is concerned with being critically reflective and considering when a change in practice is required. Single loop learning involves reactions to certain stimuli that are fairly static; double loop learning enables error detection and change through critical scrutiny. Professional reflection should facilitate defensible change where that is necessary and beneficial.

Activity 10.5   *Reflection*

How would you market yourself now for an interview? If you already have a portfolio, would you feel comfortable to share it in a job interview or do you think that it needs improvement? Your audience will need to be able to identify the most important evidence within the portfolio quickly and easily. What do you think that a potential employer will be looking for within your portfolio? Who might help you to prepare for that?

An outline answer is provided at the end of the chapter.

Chapter summary

This chapter has considered the importance of the professional portfolio and also what should be included in it, related to some of the relevant professional expectations requiring this (NMC, 2008c). The quality, presentation and content of the portfolio are all equally important. We have suggested portfolio content such as analysing and appraising personal strengths, learning needs and even contemplating barriers to that learning. Keeping this resource neat will further demonstrate high standards of documentation skills and reinforce the need for good organisational skills in theory and practice – at the university and during placements. It is also vital to remember that the portfolio should be judged by the quality of the work you have created and compiled, and not by the quantity of paper that you have included in it.

Activities: Brief outline answers

Activity 10.2 (page 199)

Why would Julian benefit from the use of a portfolio? If he has an ongoing record of learning achievement with him, he will be able to show his current mentor what he was signed off as having achieved in his first placement. His first mentor may well have also provided comments evaluating Julian's performance overall. From this record the current mentor may glean how much he has achieved so far and what his overall level of aptitude is. As each mentor is an individually accountable practitioner, they should trust each other to make effective judgements. The current mentor might still supervise 'from a distance' to make sure Julian is maintaining skills already signed off, but effectively they should enable Julian to progress. So the record should act as an evidential resource, helping to prevent unnecessary duplication of effort for all concerned.

Activity 10.4 (page 203)

Staff Nurse Bauby needs to adequately prepare for the future interview process she will have to go through. A potential employer will be looking for a candidate who has the appropriate skills to effectively do the job they have applied for. They might also be looking for a candidate who can demonstrate that they are creative, flexible, open to new ideas and willing to work hard. Organisational skills, good interpersonal skills and the ability to learn from mistakes might also be regarded as prioritised attributes. Personal qualities and organisational flair will, of course, need to be underpinned by the appropriate qualifications and experience. There will be both essential and desirable requirements of potential post holders. When looking for jobs, Staff Nurse Bauby will need the essential requirements to apply, but it will clearly be advantageous also to have all or some of the desirable ones.

Activity 10.5 (page 210)

How the portfolio might help you to sell yourself:

- Professional regulation: the NMC expects you to evidence your lifelong learning and development in this way and a potential employer may ask to see the portfolio to check that you are complying with this.
- Evidence-based practice: all professionals need to be able to articulate defensible evidence supporting their practice, ensuring that it is safe; this commitment could also be demonstrated in the portfolio.
- Evidencing development through written reflective account: demonstrating evidence of lifelong learning.

Who might help you with this resource?

* Personal tutor
* Mentors
* Royal College of Nursing
* Enquiry-based learning facilitators

You should feel increasingly confident that you can effectively market yourself by knowing where to look for learning opportunities and following them up in a professional manner. You need to be very clear of any potential employer's expectations of you should you apply for a job, so familiarising yourself with them and the job specification is critical. You should prepare for what an interviewer might ask you and look well presented and organised when you meet them. Taking in a professionally presented portfolio should be a distinct advantage.

Further reading

Luft, J and Ingham, H (1955) The Johari Window: a graphic model of interpersonal awareness. *Proceedings of the Western Training Laboratory in Group Development*. Los Angeles: UCLA.

Offers additional insight into the potential application of this interesting and useful tool.

NMC (2008) *The Code*. London: NMC.

Essential reading for al nursing students and NMC registrants.

NMC (2008) *The Prep Handbook*. London: NMC.

This publication sets out the NMC expectations of nurses' CPD.

Reed, S (2011) *Successful Portfolios for Nursing Students*. Exeter: Learning Matters.

Another book in the same series as this book (Transforming Nursing Practice), which provides a step-by-step guide though the process of creating a portfolio.

Useful websites

www.businessballs.com

This site contains diverse and useful examples of tools to use and specific activities that you can do in order to understand and develop yourself more.

www.RCN.org.uk

An important source of professional advice, support and guidance for both nursing students and registered nurses. You need to become a member in order to gain access to the full range of resources available.

Glossary

Bibliographic management software – a computer package that allows you to organise and store references you have accessed when, for example, researching for an assignment. In addition, you can print the references out in the referencing style your university advises.

Bookmark – when you find a web page of interest, you can mark the page so that you can return to it at a later date. In effect, you are creating a shortcut to quickly revisit the page without having to navigate the internet again.

Confounding variables – variables that are not factors being considered overtly and consciously in an observational study or experiment, but may nevertheless be influential on the outcomes. These unanticipated effects may be very problematic to the clarity of the research process.

Database application – a structured collection of records or data that is stored on a computer system. It is used to store information or data, which is broken down into records to make it easier to search and retrieve. For example, a database could contain data such as patient contact details, GP information, diagnoses, medication, consultations, etc.

Electrolytes – compounds in the blood necessary for normal cell activity.

Electronic alert – there are a number of services, including one from the British Library, which allow licensed users to set up a profile. So, whenever an article is published in the topic area you have set up within your profile, or an issue of a journal title you've identified in the profile is published, you will be sent an email alerting you to this.

Electronic devices – usually medical devices to assist in delivering a treatment or medicine to a patient.

External validity – the capacity to generalise the results of one study in one setting to other settings.

Federated search – a facility that allows you to search across a number of databases simultaneously. It is a good starting point when searching for journal articles on a topic, from where you can move on to a native database (see below) search.

Grounded theory – an inductive qualitative research design, wherein theory is generated from the data collected within the research process.

In situ – a term used to mean 'in place'

Inter-library loan system – a library service that enables you to request books or journal articles that are not held or available in the library you are using. There may be restrictions or charges on this service.

Interrogate – to ask questions. In terms of a database, you are asking for information in the form of queries and reports. For example, you might want to ask a patient database which patients have not had their treatment reassessed in the last six months.

Mail merge – a facility that allows you to make a standard form letter and merge it with a list of names and addresses to create a personalised letter for sending out. It enables you to produce hundreds of letters with a few clicks of the mouse, rather than writing a long list of individual letters.

Meta-analysis – analyses the combined results of several studies that are compatible or amenable to comparison. This is normally enabled through identification of a common measure.

Native database – rather than searching across a range of resources simultaneously, you can go to a specific or native database. This allows you to use more advanced searching techniques.

Negative fluid balance – fluid intake is less than fluid output.

Nomogram – a graphic representation of numerical values (used when calculating drug doses).

Non-experimental – a research design in which there is no use of control or comparison groups. This is often found to be qualitative research.

Positive fluid balance – fluid intake is greater than fluid output.

Pressure ulcers – injury to skin and underlying tissue as a result of pressure with or without shearing or friction.

Randomised controlled trial – a precise type of scientific experiment wherein participants are randomly allocated to either intervention or control groups, with effort made to contain confounding variables, in order to identify whether a new intervention is effective.

Sliding sheets – an aid to move patients safely – for example, up the bed.

Stratified sample – a random sample that represents specific levels of diversity within a sample (e.g. if you were interviewing nursing students you would identify how many male and female participants you would need based on estimates of how many of each are represented).

Systematic review – a very distinct type of literature review, focused on a research question and in doing so makes strenuous efforts to find all relevant evidence that meets its inclusion criteria. It is a secondary source, defined by completeness of literature searching and quality of appraisals of identified and included evidence.

Transparency of research process – the very real need for researchers to provide sufficient, relevant and meaningful information for all key stakeholders, regarding the research aims, design, conduct and findings.

Virtual learning environment – an electronic system that supports learning and is an adjunct to the face-to-face learning experience. Students are attached to their modules on the system and can access course handouts, be directed to activities and further reading. Students and staff can also engage in discussion and share information.

White coat syndrome – a term used when a patient's blood pressure reading is higher in a medical situation (for example, in a hospital ward or GP surgery) than at home.

References

Adlit.org (undated) *All About Adolescent Literacy: Resources for parents and educators of kids in grades 4–12*. Available online at www.adlit.org.

Aiken, F and Dale, C (2007) A *Review of the Literature into Dyslexia in Nursing Practice*. London: Royal College of Nursing.

Alaszewski, A (2003) The impact of the Bristol Royal Infirmary disaster and inquiry on public services in the UK. *Journal of Interprofessional Care*, 16(4): 371–378.

Arkell, S and Bayliss-Pratt, L (2007) How nursing students can make the most of placements. *Nursing Times*, 103 (20): 26–30.

Bach, S and Grant, A (2009) *Communication and Interpersonal Skills for Nurses*. Exeter: Learning Matters.

Bandman, EL and Bandman, B (1995) *Critical Thinking in Nursing* (2nd edition). Norwalk, CT: Appleton and Lange.

BAPEN (2003) *Malnutrition Universal Screening Tool*. Available online at www.bapen.org.uk/pdfs/must/must_full.pdf (accessed 12 December 2010).

Benner, P (1984) *From Novice to Expert: Excellence and power in clinical nursing practice*. Menlo Park, California: Addison Wesley Publishing.

BNF (2010) *BNF 60*. Available online at www.bnf.org/bnf (accessed 12 December 2010).

Boulos, MNK, Maramba, I and Wheeler, S (2006) Wikis, blogs and podcasts: a new generation of web-based tools for virtual collaborative clinical practice and education. *BMC Medical Education*, 6.

Brosnan, M, Evans, W, Brosnan, E and Brown, G (2006) Implementing objective structured clinical skills evaluation (OSCE) in nurse registration programmes in a centre in Ireland: a utilisation focused evaluation. *Nurse Education Today*, 26: 115–122.

Burnard, P (1995) *Learning Human Skills: A guide for nurses* (3rd edition). Oxford: Heinemann.

Carper, B (1978) Fundamental patterns of knowing in nursing. *Advances in Nursing Science*, 1(1): 13–23.

Castledine, G and Close, A (eds) (2007) *Oxford Handbook of General Adult Nursing*. Oxford: Oxford University Press.

CILIP (2010) *Information Literacy: The skills*. Available online at www.cilip.org.uk/get-involved/advocacy/learning/information-literacy/pages/skills.aspx (accessed 21 September 2010).

Clark, A (2009) *Capturing Learning in Practice from Practice: Case study for the Centre of Integrated Learning, University of Nottingham*. Internal publication available online at www.nottingham.ac.uk/integrativelearning.

Clouder, L (2003) Becoming professional: exploring the complexities of professional socialization in health and social care. *Learning in Health & Social Care*, 2 (4): 213–222.

Clouder, L and Sellers, J (2004) Reflective practice and clinical supervision: an interprofessional perspective. *Journal of Advanced Nursing*, 46 (3): 262–269.

Cottrell, S (2003) *The Study Skills Handbook* (2nd edition). Hampshire: Palgrave Macmillan.

Davies, C (2010) I want to spend a penny, not go to the shop: nurses to be taught euphemisms, in *Guardian*, 20 August 2010. Available online at www.guardian.co.uk (accessed 6 September 2010).

Deigham, G (2008) Foreign guide t'speak Yorkshire, on *Sky News Online*, 8 August 2008 (accessed 6 September 2010)

Department of Education (2010) *National Curriculum Assessments at Key Stage 2 in England*. London: National Statistics Office.

Department of Health (1997) *The New NHS: Modern, dependable*. London: The Stationery Office.

Department of Health (1998) *A First Class Service: Quality in the NHS*. London: The Stationery Office.

Department of Health (1999a) *Making a Difference: Strengthening the nursing, midwifery and health visiting contribution to health and healthcare*. London: The Stationery Office.

Department of Health (1999b) *Saving Lives: Our healthier nation*. London: The Stationery Office.

Department of Health (2000) *The NHS Plan: A plan for investment, a plan for reform*. London: The Stationery Office.

Department of Health (2001) *Essence of Care*. London: HMSO.

Department of Health (2003) *Toolkit for Producing Patient Information* (Version 2). London: Department of Health.

Department of Health (2005) *Mental Capacity Act, 2005*. Available online at www.opsi.gov.uk/acts/acts2007a.htm (accessed 5 March 2010).

Department of Health (2006) *Chief Nursing Officer's Review of Mental Health Nursing: Summary of responses to the consultation*. London: HMSO.

Department of Health (2007) *Transfer of Information Across the Interface between Health Care Professionals and Other Agencies*. London: Department of Health.

Department of Health (2008a) Evaluation of information prescriptions. *London: Department of Health*.

Department of Health (2008b) *High Quality for All: NHS next stage review, final (Darzi) report*. London: HMSO.

Department of Health (2010) *Essence of Care 2010: Benchmarks for the fundamental aspects of care*. London: The Stationery Office. Available online at www.tsoshop.co.uk (accessed 7 November 2010).

Dimond, B (2008) *Legal Aspects of Nursing* (5th edition). Essex: Longman.

Driscoll, J and Teh, B (2001) The potential of reflective practice to develop individual orthopaedic nurse practitioners and their practice. *Journal of Orthopaedic Nursing*, 5: 95–103.

Driscoll, JJ (2007) Chapter 2: Supported reflective learning: the essence of clinical supervision?, in Driscoll, JJ (ed.) *Practising Clinical Supervision: A reflective approach for healthcare professionals* (2nd edition). Edinburgh: Bailliere Tindall, Elsevier.

Easton, P, Entwistle, A and Williams, B (2010) Health in the 'hidden population' of people with low literacy: a systematic review of the literature. *Public Health*, 2010, 10: 459. Available online at www.biomedcentral.com/content/pdf/1471-2458-10-459.pdf (accessed October 2010).

Edwards, S (1998) Critical thinking and analysis: a model for written assignments. *British Journal of Nursing*, 7 (3): 159–165.

Ewles, L and Simnet, I (2003) *Promoting Health: A practical guide* (5th edition). Edinburgh: Balliere and Tindall.

Flynn, R (2004) 'Soft bureacracy', governmentality and clinical governance: theoretical approaches to emergent policy, in Gray, A and Harrison, S (2004) *Governing Medicine, Theory and Practice*. Berkshire: Open University Press.

The Focus Group UK (2007) *Lay Representatives Focus Group Consultation Report On General Entry Requirements to Pre-registration Nursing and Midwifery Education on behalf of the Nursing and Midwifery Council, October 2007*. Available online at www.nmc-uk.org/Documents/Consultations (accessed October 2010). London: NMC.

Gibbs, G (1988) *Learning by Doing: A guide to teaching and learning methods.* Oxford: Further Education Unit, Oxford Brookes University.

Godwin, P (2009) Information literacy: as endorsed by Barak Obama and UNESCO. *SCONUL Focus* 48: 7–9.

Goleman, D (2001) *Working with Emotional Intelligence.* London: Bloomsbury Publishing.

Goodman, B and Clemow, R (2008) *Nursing and Working with Other People.* Exeter: Learning Matters.

The Health and Social Care Information Centre (2010) *NHS: The Information Centre for Health and Social Care: statistics on obesity, physical activity and diet: England, 2010.* Available online at www.ic.nhs.uk/webfiles/publications/opad10/Statistics_on_Obesity_Physical_Activity_and_Diet_England_2010.pdf (accessed 13 November 2010).

Hogan, M, Bolten, S, Ricci, M and Taliaferro, D (2008) *Nursing Fundamentals.* New Jersey: Prentice Hall.

Hubley, J and Copeman, J (2008) *Practical Health Promotion.* Cambridge: Polity Press.

Johns, C (1996) Visualizing and realizing caring in practice through guided reflection. *Journal of Advanced Nursing*, 24(6): 1135–1143.

Johns, C (2004) *Becoming a Reflective Practitioner* (2nd edition). Oxford: Blackwell.

Johns, C (2006) *Engaging Reflection in Practice.* Oxford: Wiley Blackwell.

Johnson, M, Jefferies, D and Langdon, R (2010) The Nursing and Midwifery Content Audit Tool (nmcat): a short nursing documentation audit tool. *Journal of Nursing Management*, 18 (7): 832–45, October.

Jones, SA and Brown, L (1991) Critical thinking: impact of nursing education. *Journal of Advanced Nursing*, 16, 529–533.

Krischke, MM (2009) *Avoiding Nurses' Biggest Communication Mistakes*, Nursing News in NurseZone.com at www.nursezone.com/nursing-news-events/more-news/Avoiding-Nurses-Biggest-Communication-Mistakes_32566.aspx (accessed October 2010).

Law, L, Akroyd, K and Burke, L (2010) Improving nurse documentation and record keeping in stoma care. *British Journal of Nursing*, 19(21): 1328–1332.

Lees, L (2010) Improving the quality of nursing documentation on an acute medicine unit. *Nursing Times*, 106(37): 22–26, 21 September.

Longley, M, Shaw, C and Dolan, G (2007) *Nursing: Towards 2015.* Available online at www.nmc-uk.org (accessed 14 October 2010).

Lowthian, P (1987) The practical assessment of pressure sore risk. *Care–Science and Practice*, 5(4): 3–7.

Luettal, D and Bischler, A (2010) Safety when giving insulin in hospital. *Nursing Times*, 106 (39): 12–13

Luft, J and Ingham, H (1955) The Johari Window: a graphic model of interpersonal awareness. *Proceedings of the Western Training Laboratory in Group Development.* Los Angeles: UCLA.

Maddex, S (2009) Measuring vital signs, in Baillie, L (2009) *Developing Practical Adult Nursing Skills* (3rd edition). London: Hodder Arnold.

Medical Devices Agency (2003) *Infusion Systems.* Available online at www.mhra.gov.uk (accessed 28 November 2010).

Melia, K (1987) *Learning and Working: The occupational socialisation of nurses.* London: Tavistock Publications.

Millard, L, Hallett, C and Luker, K (2006) Nurse–patient interaction and decision-making in care: patient involvement in community nursing. *Journal of Advanced Nursing*, 55(2): 142–150.

Mosteller, RD (1987) Simplified calculation of body surface area. *New England Journal of Medicine*, 317: 1098.

National Academy of Science (1996) *National Science Education Standards*. Available online at www.nap.edu/readingroom/books/nses and www.literacynet.org/science/scientificliteracy.html (accessed 6 September 2010).

National Health Service (undated) *An Easy Guide To Breast Screening: A leaflet by and for women with learning disabilities*. London: Department of Health.

Norton, D, McLaren, R and Exton-Smith, AN (1975) *An Investigation of Geriatric Problems in Hospital*. London: Churchill Livingstone.

Nottingham University Hospital (2010) *Health Record Keeping Policy* (Version 2) 3 March (NUH internal document). Available online at www.nuh.nhs.uk/about/boardpapers/policy (accessed 16 December 2010).

Nursing and Midwifery Council (NMC) (2004) *Standards of Proficiency for Pre-registration Nursing Education*. London: NMC.

Nursing and Midwifery Council (NMC) (2007a) *Introduction of Essential Skills Clusters for Pre-registration Nursing Programmes*. London: NMC.

Nursing and Midwifery Council (NMC) (2007b) *Mapping of Essential Skills Clusters to the Standards of Proficiency for Pre-registration Nursing Education (NMC 2004) Annexe 3 to NMC Circular 07/2007* (accessed 23 August 2004).

Nursing and Midwifery Council (NMC) (2008a) *Evidence of Literacy and Numeracy Required for Entry to Pre-registration Nursing and Midwifery Programmes, Nursing and Midwifery Council Circular 03/2008*. Available online at www.nmc.org (accessed 24 August 2010).

Nursing and Midwifery Council (NMC) (2008b) *The Code: Standards of conduct, performance and ethics for nurses and midwives*. London: NMC.

Nursing and Midwifery Council (NMC) (2008c) *The Prep Handbook*. London: NMC.

Nursing and Midwifery Council (NMC) (2008d) *Standards to Support Learning and Assessment in Practice*. London: NMC.

Nursing and Midwifery Council (2009) Record keeping interview with Martine Tune. NMC News Edition 29. Available online at www.nmc-uk.org/Nurses-and-midwives/Record-keeping-interview-with-Martine-Tune (accessed October 2010).

NMC (2010a) *Guidelines for Records and Record Keeping: Guidance for nurses and midwives*. London: NMC. Available online at www.nmc.uk.org (accessed October 2010).

NMC (2010b) *Reasons for the Interim Order Panel Hearing of the Investigating Committee Panel held at 61 Aldwych, Centrium on 19 March 2010*. Available online at www.nmc.uk.org (accessed October 2010).

Nursing and Midwifery Council (NMC) (2010c) *Standards for Pre-registration Nursing Education*. London: NMC. Available online at www.nmc.uk.org (accessed October 2010).

Nursing and Midwifery Council (NMC) (2010d) *NMC Guidance on Professional Conduct for Nursing and Midwifery Students, 2010*. London: NMC.

Organisation for Economic and Cooperative Development (undated) *Adult Literacy*. Available online at www.oecd.org/document.

Parnia, S, Spearpoint, K and Fenwick, PB (2007) Near death experiences, cognitive function and psychological outcomes of surviving cardiac arrest. *Resuscitation*, 74(2): 215–221.

Pheasey, A (2002) What do adult literacy students think being literate is?, in Research in Practice in Adult Literacy (RPAC) *Network Learning at the Centre Press*, pp1–24. Available online at http://library.nald.ca (accessed October 2010).

Phillippi, JC and Buxton, M (2010) Web 2.0: easy tools for busy clinicians. *Journal of Midwifery and Women's Health*, 55(5): 472–476.

Porter, S (2008) *First Steps in Research: A pocketbook for healthcare students.* Philadelphia: Elsevier.

Protheroe, J, Nutbeam, Dl and Rowlands, J (2009) Health literacy: a necessity for increasing participation in health care. *British Journal of General Practice*, 59(567): 721–723, 1 October.

Rentschler, DD, Eaton, J, Cappiello, J, McNally, SF and McWilliam, P (2007) Evaluation of undergraduate students using objective structured clinical evaluation. *Journal of Nursing Education*, 46 (3): 140–145.

Robinson, L (2008) *Health Literacy: Do patients understand?* Wild Iris Medical Education. Available online at www.NursingCEU.com (accessed November 2010).

Rogers, CR (1957) Becoming a person, in Doniger, S (ed.) *Healing, Human and Divine.* New York: Association Press.

Rogers, CR (1980) Growing old – or older and growing. *Journal of Humanistic Psychology*, 20(4): 5–16, Fall.

Royal College of Nursing (RCN) (2005) *Clinical Practice Guidelines: Perioperative fasting in adults and children. An RCN guideline for the multidisciplinary team* (full version). London: RCN.

Royal College of Nursing (RCN) (2006). *Putting Information at the Heart of Nursing Care.* London: RCN.

Royal College of Paediatrics and Child Health (2009) *UK-WHO Growth Charts – Fact Sheet 1: What are growth charts and why do we need them?* (Available online at: www.rcpch.ac.uk/Research/Growth_Charts_Education_Training_Resources (accessed 21 November 2010).

Santry, C (2010) Nursing seen as hard, nasty and menial. *Nursing Times*, 106(42): 2–5.

Schön, DA (1983) *The Reflective Practitioner: How professionals think in action.* New York: Basic Books.

Schön, DA (1987) *Educating the Reflective Practitioner*, to the 1987 meeting of the American Educational Research Association, Washington, DC.

SCONUL (2007*) Information Skills in Higher Education: A SCONUL position paper.* Available online at www.sconul.ac.uk/groups/information_literacy/papers/Seven_pillars.html (accessed 21 September 2010).

Scott, O (2009) *Full Blood Count.* Available online at www.patient.co.uk/doctor/Full-Blood-Count.htm (accessed 11 December 2010).

Shaffer, SC, Lackey, SP and Bolling, GW (May/June 2006) Blogging as a venue for nurse faculty development. *Nursing Education Perspectives*, 126–129.

Sharples, K (2009) *Learning to Learn in Nursing Practice.* Exeter: Learning Matters.

Sharples, K (2011) *Successful Practice Learning for Nursing Students* (2nd edition of *Learning to Learn in Nursing Practice*). Exeter: Learning Matters.

Shaw, A, Ibrahim, S, Reid, F, Usher, M and Rowlands, G (2009) Patients' perspectives of the doctor–patient relationship and information giving across a range of literacy levels. *Patient Education and Counselling*, 75(1): 114–120, April.

Shears, R (2010) British nurse told to take English test before she can work in Australia, *Mail Online World News,* 6 September.

Spouse, J (2000) An impossible dream? Images of nursing held by pre-registration students and their effect on sustaining motivation to become nurses. *Journal of Advanced Nursing*, 32(3): 730–739.

Starkings, S and Krause, L (2010) *Passing Calculations Tests for Nursing Students.* Exeter: Learning Matters.

Sully, P and Dallas, J (2005) *Essential Communication Skills for Nursing.* London: Elsevier Mosby.

Summers, S and Summers, H (2010) Tackle harmful media stereotypes by advocating for the profession. *Nursing Times*, 106(41): 9.

Surgical Tutor (2010) *Fluid and Electrolyte Balance*. Available online at www.surgical-tutor.org.uk (accessed 5 November 2010).

Swannell, J (ed.) (1986) *The Little Oxford Dictionary of Current English*, 6th edition. Oxford: Clarendon Press.

Taylor, BJ (2006) *Reflective Practice: A Guide for Nurses and Midwives* (2nd edition). Berkshire: Open University Press.

Temple, M (2005) *Grammar Book*. Oxford: Blackwell.

The Plain English Campaign (2010) *How to Write in Plain English*. Available online at www.plainenglish.co.uk.

Thornton, P (2002) *The Triangles of Management and Leadership*. Coral Springs, Florida: Llumina Press.

Titchen, A (2000) *Professional Craft Knowledge in Patient-Centred Nursing and the Facilitation of its Development*. D.Phil. thesis (1999), Linacre College. Oxford: Ashdale.

Wagner, C, Semmler, C, Good, A, Wardle, J (2009) Health literacy and self-efficacy for participating in colorectal cancer screening: the role of information processing. *Patient Education and Counselling*, 3: 352–357, June.

Walsh, M, Bailey, PH and Koren, I (2009) Objective structured clinical evaluation of clinical competence and integrative review. *Journal of Advanced Nursing*, 65 (8): 1584–1595.

Walton, G, Childs, S and Blenkinsopp, E (2005) Using mobile technologies to give health students access to learning resources in the UK community setting. *Health Information and Libraries Journal*, 22 (Suppl. 2), 51–65.

Waterlow, J (1985) Pressure sores: a risk assessment card. *Nursing Times*, 81(48).

Weir-Hughes, D (2010) New education standards give clarity to nurse's role. *Nursing Times*, 106: 42.

Whitcombe, SW (2005) Understanding healthcare from sociological perspectives, in Clouston, T J and Weston, L (2005) *Working in Health and Social Care*. London: Elsevier.

White, D, Schelten, S, Kelly, B and Casey, P (2010) Written information on bipolar affective disorder: the patients' perspective. *The Psychiatrist*, 34: 418–422.

Williamson, GR, Jenkinson, T and Proctor-Childs, T (2008) *Nursing in Comtemporary Healthcare Practice*. Exeter: Learning Matters.

Willis, DS, Kennedy, CM and Kilbride, L (2008) Breast cancer screening in women with learning disabilities: current knowledge and considerations. *British Journal of Learning Disabilities*, 36(3): 171–184.

Witherington, EMA, Pirzada, OM and Avery, AJ (2007) Communication gaps and readmissions to hospital for patients aged 75 years and older: observational study. *Quality and Safety in Health Care*, 2008, 17: 71–75.

World, H (2004) *Lost in Translation: Nurses trained to be sensitive to cultural and linguistic differences help improve access to care for non-English-speaking patients*. Available online at www.nurseweek.com/news/Features/04-08/LinguisticDifferences.asp (accessed 6 September 2010).

Younger, P (2010) Using wikis as an online health information resource. *Nursing Standard*, 24(36): 49–56.

Zurmehly, J (2010) Personal Digital Assistants (PDAs): review and evaluation. *Nursing Education Perspectives*, 31(3): 179–182.

Index